SOCCER
SMARTS
FOR KIDS

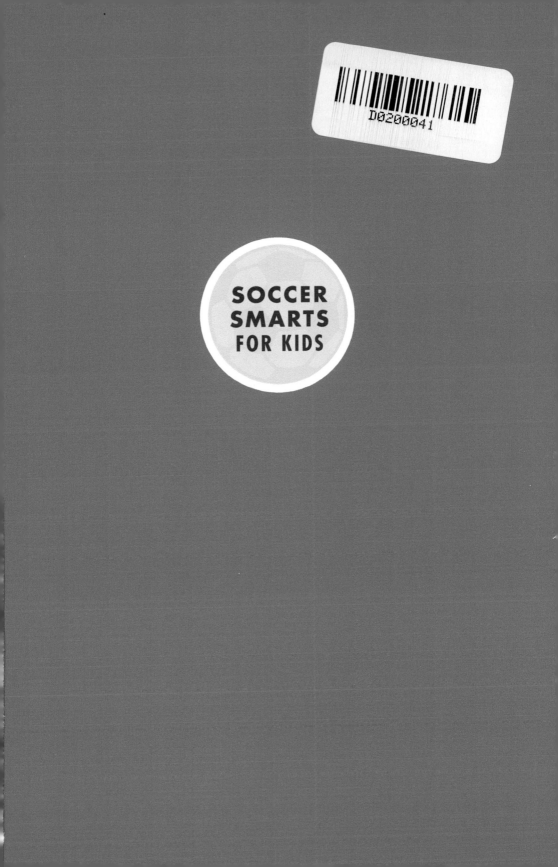

For general information on our other products and services or to obtain technical support, please contact our Customer Care Department within the United States at (866) 744-2665, or outside the United States at (510) 253-0500.

Rockridge Press publishes its books in a variety of electronic and print formats. Some content that appears in print may not be available in electronic books, and vice versa.

Illustrations: Sam Ledoyen © 2016

Front cover photograph © XiXinXing/Shutterstock; Interior photographs © Photo Works/Shutterstock, p. 32; Jeff McIntosh/Associated Press, p. 56; Armando Franca/Associated Press, p. 84; Matthew Pearce/Associated Press, p. 96; Brynn Anderson/Associated Press, p. 116; Marcos Mesa Sam Wordley / Shutterstock, p. 142

ISBN Softcover 978-1-62315-690-9 | eBook 978-1-62315-691-6

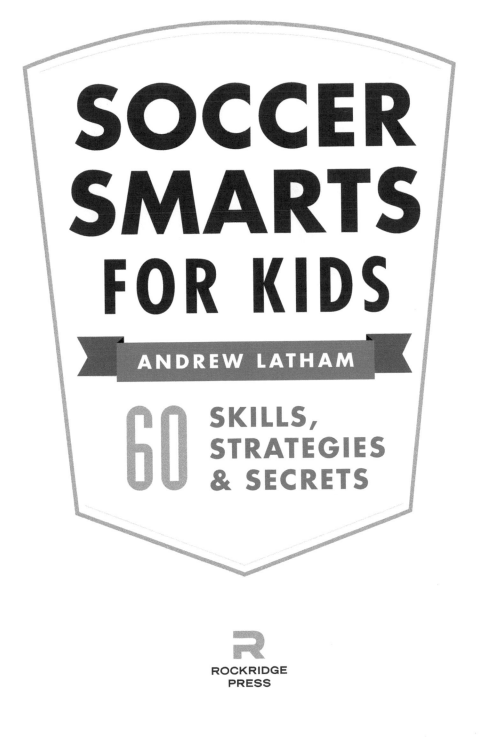

SOCCER SMARTS FOR KIDS

ANDREW LATHAM

60 SKILLS, STRATEGIES & SECRETS

ROCKRIDGE PRESS

CONTENTS

Introduction 8

PLAYBOOK 11

SKILLS 🥾

1 Receive the Ball 20

2 Receive a Pass 22

3 Use Your Thighs and Chest 24

4 Make Short-Range Passes 26

5 Make Mid-Range Passes 29

★ **DAVID BECKHAM** 32

6 Make Long-Distance Passes 34

7 Bend the Ball: Inside 36

8 Chip the Ball 39

9 Strike on a Volley 42

10 Take a Penalty 44

11 Shield the Ball 46

12 Juggle the Ball 48

13 Play with Both Feet 50

14 Shoot from Inside the Box 52

15 Shoot against the Keeper 54

★ **CHRISTINE SINCLAIR** 56

16 Bend the Ball: Outside 58

17 Head the Ball. 61

STRATEGIES ⚽

1 Learn by Watching 64

2 Remember and Predict Patterns. 67

3 Be Aware of Your Space 70

4 Receive a Pass. 73

5 Stay Onside 75

6 What to Do in Wide Positions 78

7 Get Behind the Ball 81

★ **MIA HAMM**. 84

8 Take a Throw-In 86

9 Receive a Throw-In 88

10 Know Common Patterns 90

11 Keep the Ball or Pass It? 93

★ **LIONEL MESSI** 96

12 Get Past the Other Team 98

13 Beat a Player without Touching the Ball. 103

14 Choose the Right Pass 105

15 Help the Player on the Ball 109

16 Help Your Team Defend. 113

★ ALEX MORGAN 116

17 Understand the Back Line 118

18 Cross the Ball. 123

19 Defend the Cross. 127

20 Create Space. 130

21 Break Their Lines. 133

22 Live in the Triangle 138

★ CRISTIANO RONALDO 142

23 What to Do 1 vs. 1 144

24 Get the Ball Back 147

25 Work Together on the Back Line 150

26 Get to the Arriving Triangle. 153

27 Get Ready to Score 156

FOR PARENTS

What Is Success? 160

Encourage Practice 162

The Role You Play 163

At the Game. 164

Showing Support 165

Acknowledgments 167

Index 168

INTRODUCTION

Hello, soccer player!

This book has one purpose: to give you the tools to become the best soccer player you can be.

When I was a young player, I thought my coaches were the ones who decided how far I could go. When I became older, I realized I was the one who held the keys to my development as a soccer player. I just didn't know where my keys were! Think of this book as your keys and instruction manual.

Every soccer player is an individual. Although soccer is a team sport, it's a team sport that relies on lots of individual actions. Soccer players are unique, and no two players develop at the same pace. We all have different periods of growth. The one thing we all need is great technique.

There is no "special secret" to becoming a top athlete other than hard work. If you work hard and practice your technique, you will develop your talent. In soccer we say, "talent beats hard work when talent works hard." This means that if you have talent and you work hard at developing your skills, you become unbeatable. We usually see top players scoring goals or making game-winning tackles, but what we don't see is how hard they work in practice.

When you practice with your team or friends, remember to have fun! You naturally want to win, score goals, and make passes, but it is more important to enjoy yourself and have fun. If it's not fun, you will eventually stop playing and move on to another activity. If you watch the best soccer players in the world, you will see that they are having fun and enjoy being on a team with their teammates.

Most soccer experts agree that there four pieces to the soccer jigsaw puzzle: technical ability, tactical understanding, physical ability, and the psychological part of the game. This book highlights fundamental skills and specific strategies to develop these four pieces, as well as coaches' secrets for excelling at the game.

In this book, you will learn some drills to help you develop your technical skills. You can practice these drills on your own or with your teammates. We will also introduce you to some mental skills for becoming a smarter player and a more effective member of the team. The secrets hidden throughout this book will give you helpful tips on goal setting, physical fitness, nutrition, and preparing for practices and games. In addition, you'll meet six superstar soccer players who have all the attributes and qualities of top-level athletes. You'll even find information for your parents. Your parents are your biggest supporters, and we want to help them help you become the best player you can be.

You will see your soccer ability grow dramatically when you focus on the skills, strategies, and secrets outlined in this book and follow the examples of the featured superstars. As you improve, you'll enjoy the game even more. If you have passion for soccer and enjoy it, you'll be able to enjoy playing throughout your lifetime. You may even make it to the World Cup! ⚽

PLAYBOOK

PLAYBOOK

Soccer has a language all its own. As a player, you want to have a basic understanding of the terms and phrases that are used in the game. This way you'll know what your coach is talking about. Remember, the coach is there to help. If you hear a new word, ask what it means!

Positions

Forward (Attacker)
The forward's job is to score goals and to create more chances to score goals. If you don't buy a lottery ticket, then you can't win the big prize. In soccer, you win the big prize every time you score a goal. If you are a forward (your coach might also call you an attacker), you should be ready to help get the ball back from the other team. But your main job is trying to score goals.

Defender
The defender's most important job is to work with the goalkeeper to make sure no goals get scored. The best way

Positions

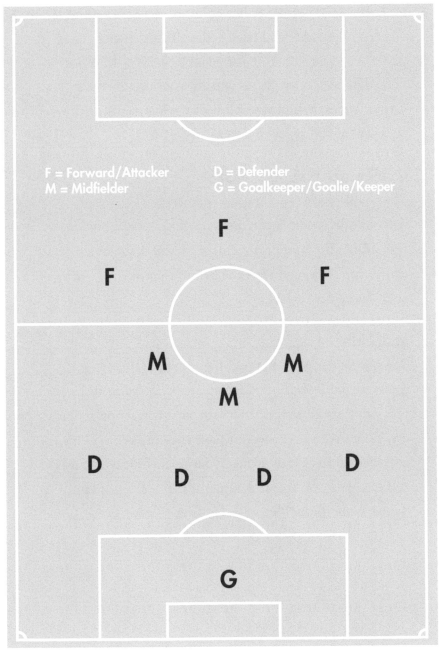

F = Forward/Attacker   D = Defender
M = Midfielder   G = Goalkeeper/Goalie/Keeper

to do this is to get the ball away from the other team. If you are a defender, you need to be able to challenge the player with the ball. You also need to work with other defenders to take space away from your opponent. Center backs, half backs, full backs, wing backs, and sweepers are all types of defenders.

Goalkeeper (Keeper/Goalie)

The goalkeeper's most important job is to keep the ball out of the net! If you are a goalkeeper, you are also responsible for communicating with the defenders on your team. When you get the ball, it's up to you to start your team's next attack.

Midfielder

The midfielder plays many different roles. If you are a midfielder and your team has the ball, you need to help move to the ball to link your attackers with your defenders. When your team doesn't have the ball, you will try to win the ball back and protect your goal. Your coach might call your position the attacking midfielder, central midfielder, wide midfielder, or defending midfielder.

Soccer Terms

above the ball: Ahead of the ball or past the ball. The area closer to the opponent's goal than the ball.

attack: When your team is going toward the opponent's goal with the ball.

back four: The defenders on a soccer team. Usually there are four of them.

below the ball: The area closer to your goal than the ball when your team is in possession.

breakaway: When you move fast with the ball toward the opponent's goal.

break the line: Getting past the imaginary line between the players on the other team.

control: When you have the ball in front of you and you can decide what to do next.

cues: Things you see in the game that tell you what is happening next.

down the field: The area between you and your team's goal.

drop down: Move down the field and behind the ball to offer support to the ball carrier.

far post: The post that is farthest away from the ball. This changes when the ball goes across the field.

front foot: The closest foot to the opponent's goal.

heavy pass: A heavy pass reaches its target with speed and power.

higher up the field: Moving up the field toward the opponent's goal.

light pass: A light pass only just gets to its target.

marking: Matching up against a player from the other team.

one-touch pass: Touching the ball with your foot only once to send it to a teammate.

support: Moving to a position on the field that helps your teammate who has the ball.

under pressure: When a player from the other team challenges you for the ball.

The Field

closed space: An area of the field that is occupied by a player from the other team.

down low or low down: A position behind the ball (close to your own goal) that allows you to support the ball carrier.

open space: An area of the field that does not have anyone from the other team in it.

safe space: The space near you that is farthest away from the nearest defender.

Play

corner: When your team is attacking and a player from the other team puts the ball out of play on their end line.

foul: When the referee decides that a player has played unfairly.

free kick: When the referee calls a foul against one team, the other team gets a free kick to restart the game.

goal: When the whole ball crosses the goal line between the goal posts.

goal kick: When one team kicks the ball over the goal line, the other team gets a special kind of free kick called a goal kick.

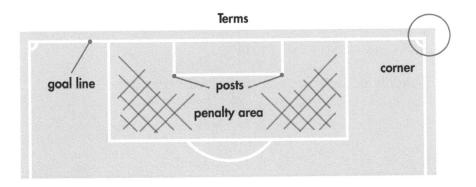

Terms

goal line

posts

penalty area

corner

offside: A player is in an offside position when he or she is in the opponents' half of the field and closer to the opponents' goal line than both the ball and the second-to-last opponent. (Most of the time, the last defensive player is the one in front of the goalkeeper.)

penalty kick: When a foul is called against the defending team in the penalty area, the attacking team gets a special kind of free kick called a penalty kick.

throw-in: When one team kicks the ball out of play on the sidelines, the other team gets to take the ball and throw it back into play.

Types of Skills and Strategies

Defending: Protecting your goal by trying to get the ball back from your opponent.

Dribbling: Touching the ball quickly to make a defender lose balance.

Passing: Kicking the ball to another player on your team.

Running: Running with the ball under control and touching it every 3 or 4 strides.

Shooting: Trying to kick the ball past the opponent's goalkeeper and into the goal.

SKILLS

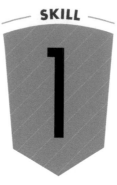

Receive the Ball

» *Passing*

There are three key points that will help you develop your ability to receive the ball. First, you have to make space and get set to receive the ball from a teammate. Second, decide what part of the body you will use to receive the ball, and where your safe space will be. Finally, before you receive the ball, you should know what you are going to do with it next. The best soccer players always make early decisions so they don't get caught with the ball!

Before you receive the pass, get into a space where your teammate can see you, so there is a clear line between you and the player with the ball. This will give your teammate the confidence to make the pass to you. Give him or her a signal to pass the ball to you and get ready for the pass.

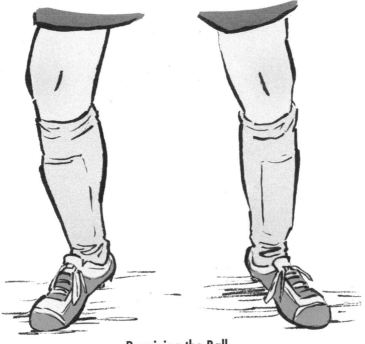

Receiving the Ball

When you receive the pass, start on your toes with your left foot pointing at ten o'clock and your right foot pointing at two o'clock. This will help you receive the ball with either foot and give you more options for your first touch. As the ball is coming to you, sneak a peek and look for your next move. When you make contact with the ball, relax your ankle joint to cushion the ball into your safe space. This is an area just in front of you in the direction that you want to go and also away from your opponents.

Now that you have the ball under control, you can make your move. Remember these three points, in order, and this will help you keep possession of the ball.

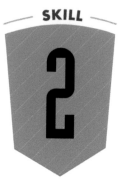

— SKILL —

Receive a Pass

» *Passing*

Your focus with this technique is to change your body position before the ball comes to you or, even better, as the ball is coming to you. Instead of having your hips both face the player who is passing you the ball, move one of your feet back so one of your shoulders is pointing in the direction the ball is coming and the other shoulder is pointing in the opposite direction. Your coach might call this position "opened up," "side on," or "half turned." It is less important what it is called and more important you understand what it means and can use the same language as your coach.

When you are in position, have the confidence to let the ball go past your feet and body and control the ball with your front foot. Keep sneaking a peek so you know what you are going to do before you get the ball, just like the world's best players. If you can't keep going forward, then you can bring the ball back into the safe space directly in front of you and keep possession.

The benefit of receiving the ball on the front foot is that you are ready to go forward if it is possible. When you receive the ball with your hips facing where the ball has come from, it's harder for you to keep the ball going forward. When you watch the top players on television, watch how often they receive the ball on their front foot.

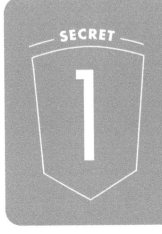

SECRET

1

RESPECT THE GAME

Always show respect to teammates, officials, and your opponents. Fair play and respect are important parts of the game.

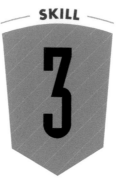

Use Your Thighs and Chest

» *Practice with friends*

The ball doesn't always come to you on the ground or high up in the air. When it comes toward you between your feet and head, there are two body parts you can use to control the ball: your thigh and your chest.

Using different parts of the body to control the ball is something good players appear to do naturally. The truth is that they practice this technique a lot.

When you control the ball with your thigh, use the right part of the thigh area or you won't be able to get the next touch on the ball. When you juggle with your thighs, use the central area. In a game, use the area just behind the knee before the start of the thigh muscle. This part of the thigh will help you move the ball into the space where you want it to go, and help you get the ball to the ground quickly so you can keep things moving.

When you chest the ball, get your chin up and out of the way and push your shoulders back to make a bigger target. As you make contact with the ball, move your chest inward and slightly bend your knees to get the ball to the ground as quickly as possible.

DRILL

Start practicing using your thigh and chest with a partner. Let him or her throw the ball to you from 10 yards away. When you are practicing this technique, always make sure you are moving toward the ball so you become comfortable judging its flight.

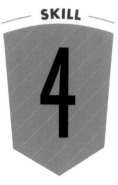

Make Short-Range Passes

» Passing

You can practice this technique with a friend, or if you can find a wall to kick the ball at, you can practice this skill yourself. The distance of this pass is between 5 and 15 yards, and the focus is on accuracy.

For this pass, use the side of your foot because it's the biggest area you can use to connect with the ball. This big area should help you make an accurate pass, and you want to keep the ball on the ground so it's easier to control the pass.

Start with the ball completely stopped. Place your nonkicking foot at the side of the ball, pointing at the target with your toe just ahead of the ball. Open up your

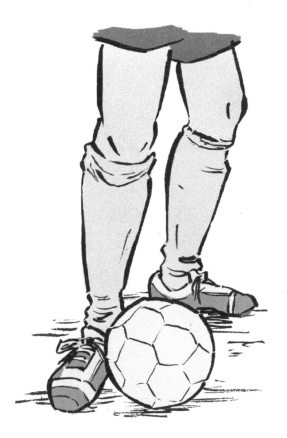

Side Foot

kicking foot so the side of your foot hits the ball. Your toe should be slightly raised with your heel down. At the point of contact, lock your ankle and raise your foot a little so you hit through the center of the ball and it stays on the ground. At the same time, try to get your chin over the ball. This also helps keep the ball on the ground.

Practice landing on your kicking foot ahead of the non-kicking foot because this will help prepare you for your next movement and help you push through the ball.

When you can do this, you can then progress to a moving ball. Take a small touch to the side to get the ball out of your feet and follow the same rules.

With this technique, your focus is on accuracy because you want to help your teammate receive the ball. Locking your ankle with your toes up and heel down will help you make the best pass possible.

COOL DOWN

At the end of each practice and each game, take some time to cool down your body and muscles. Do a light jog. Stretch your legs.

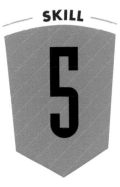

Make Mid-Range Passes

» *Passing*

We use a mid-range pass for a distance of 15 to 25 yards. A side-foot pass doesn't have the power to make it that far without marking the player who receives the ball. You can practice this skill on your own or with a partner. Start with a ball that isn't moving, so you can focus on the technique and buildup from there.

Place your nonkicking foot at the side of the ball with your toes ahead of the ball. For this pass, your plant foot needs to be a little farther away because you need more room to open up your hips when you hit the ball. You will be striking the ball with your laces. The key area is the

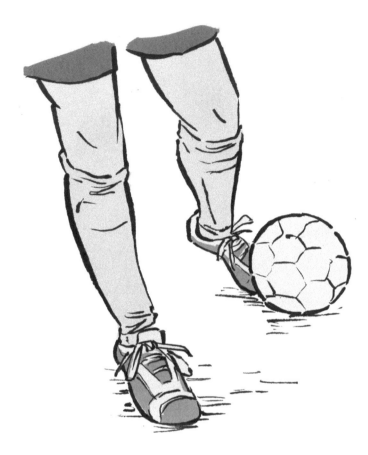

Instep Pass

knuckle on your big toe to about halfway up your instep, with your toe down and your heel up.

On contact, get your chin on your chest so you can see the ball as you hit through it. Make sure you lock your ankle. After you hit the ball, land on your kicking foot in line with, or slightly across, your nonkicking foot. By staying upright, you are keeping the ball on the ground, which makes it easier for the player receiving the pass to control the ball. Make sure you connect with the ball through the center of the ball so it doesn't spin or go in the air.

Now, try this with a moving ball. Roll the ball out to the side, get your nonkicking foot in the right place, and follow the same steps. Learning this technique is all about trial and error, so take time to practice as often as possible.

Here's a quick tip: If you hook the ball, your nonkicking foot was probably too close to the ball. If you slice the ball, your nonkicking foot was probably too far away.

David Beckham

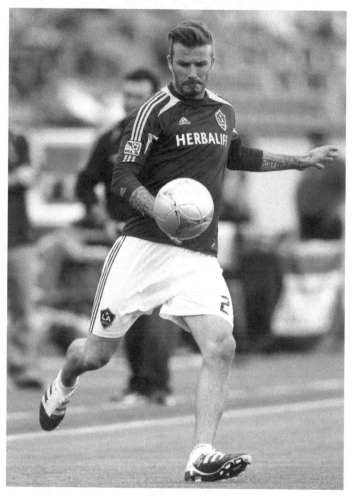

BORN: May 2, 1975 **POSITION:** Midfielder
TEAM: Manchester United, Preston North End, Real Madrid, A.C. Milan, LA Galaxy, Paris Saint-Germain, and the England national team

DAVID BECKHAM PLAYED FOR SOME of the biggest clubs in the world: Manchester United in England, A.C. Milan in Italy, and Paris Saint-Germain in France. He was also a galáctico (superstar) with Real Madrid in Spain.

There is no question that David Beckham had talent and a remarkable right foot, but his incredible work ethic was what set him apart from most players. From a very early age, Beckham wanted to play for Manchester United, and he spent hours practicing and playing to achieve his dream. When he became a professional player, he continued to spend extra time after his training sessions practicing what would become his greatest talent: striking the ball. Beckham scored many goals from free kicks and made many assists from crosses, not only because of his talent but also because he spent extra hours practicing.

Beckham also had great strength of character, which helped him through the hardest part of his career and made him a superstar. In the 1998 World Cup in France, England lost on penalties to Argentina, and Beckham was "sent off," or made to leave the field. Many of the fans in England blamed Beckham for the defeat, and he was booed by the fans in England when he played for Manchester United. He was also booed by many England fans when he played for the national team.

This made Beckham work harder and harder. In 2001, he scored the goal that took England to the World Cup, and he became a hero. Many other players would not have been able to handle the pressure, but Beckham showed that hard work and talent, when combined, are unstoppable.

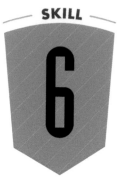

SKILL

6

Make Long-Distance Passes

» *Passing*

This type of pass is important because if you can hit a long ball accurately, you have a great range for passing. Coaches are always looking for players who can pass accurately over long distances. When you can cover a great distance with accurate passing, you are essentially making the field shorter for you and your teammates, and this gives you an advantage.

When you pass over a long distance of more than 30 yards, you almost always pass in the air. This pass is used to switch the play to the other side of the field or kick a long ball into the space behind your opponent. This type of pass needs to be accurate, or you will most likely lose possession of the ball.

Always try to practice this technique with at least one teammate so you are not wasting your time and energy chasing the ball. Start with a completely stopped ball and approach the ball from a few paces back. Your nonkicking foot is ahead of the ball and a little bit farther away from the ball because you need space to generate power in your kick. As with the mid-range pass, you are striking with your instep from the knuckle of your big toe to halfway up your instep with your toe down and your heel up.

The difference here is that you are striking the bottom half of the ball to get the ball in the air. On contact, you should be slightly leaning back, which also helps the ball go in the air. Kick through the ball. Your kicking foot should land across your body on the far side of your plant foot.

When you have mastered this skill, practice making contact with a ball that is moving. Again, learning this technique will take a lot of trial and error, but the more you practice, the better you will become.

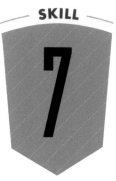

Bend the Ball: Inside

» *Passing* » *Shooting*

Bending the ball with the inside of your foot is a technique you will see a lot in games. A good free kick will bend into the top corner of the goal, away from the keeper. Corners and free kicks are good examples of this skill, but you will also use it when you cross the ball from open play and when you shoot the ball across the goal. It's a great skill to be able to do.

The key to this skill is getting your feet in the right place and making contact with the ball so you get the ball *spinning*. You can practice the technique on your own against a wall or with a friend who will be about 15 yards away. Start with a completely stopped ball.

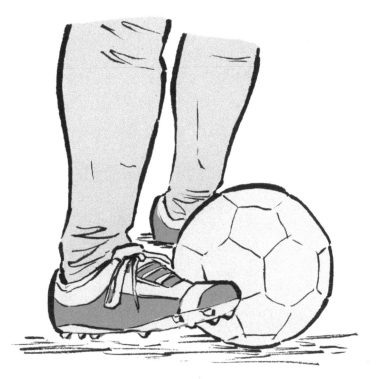

Inside of the Foot

Place your nonkicking foot at the side of the ball with your toes ahead of the ball. Hit the ball with your toes up and heel down on the outside of the ball so it starts to spin. With a *right-footed* kick, it *spins counter-clockwise*, and with a *left-footed* kick, it will *spin clockwise*. Watch the ball as it moves, look for the spin, and land on your kicking foot past your nonkicking foot. If you want to keep the ball low, make contact with the center of the ball. If you want the ball to go in the air, connect with the bottom half of the ball.

Now, try this with a moving ball. Take a touch to roll it, plant your nonkicking foot, and repeat the technique. It will take a little time to learn, but it's like riding a bike: Once you learn how to do it, you never lose it.

Go practice!

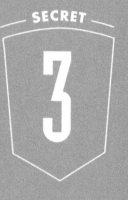

SECRET

3

TAKE NOTES

Start taking notes after practice and games. Write down what you did well, what you think you can do better, and what your coach told you at the end of the game.

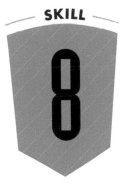
Chip the Ball

» Passing » Shooting

Chipping the ball is similar to many of the passes we have discussed. The difference is that the ball goes up in the air and then quickly to the ground. You can chip the ball over the other team's defenders and into open space. You can also chip the ball over the wall from a free kick. When you master the skill, you can chip the ball over the keeper in a 1-vs.-1 situation or from a distance if the keeper is off his or her line.

It's much easier to chip a ball rolling to you, because you can use the movement of the ball to get your foot under the ball and chip it into the air. On contact, get your nonkicking foot at the side of the ball with your toe

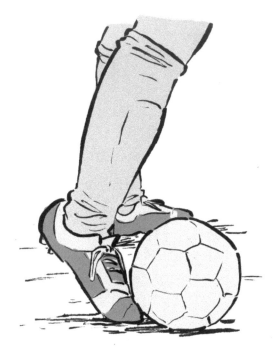

Chipping: Side View

just ahead of the ball. Point your toe down and your heel up, and try to get your foot at 45 degrees. You want to hit the bottom of the ball with the knuckle of your big toe. After you kick the ball, follow through with your kicking foot. This will put backspin on the ball, which will slow the ball down when it hits the ground.

When you have mastered this technique, try to chip the ball to a partner 20 yards away. Roll the ball to the side or ahead of you and follow the same steps. On contact, lean forward just a little bit and get your chin on your chest. This will help you get your toe underneath the ball and swipe the ball into the air.

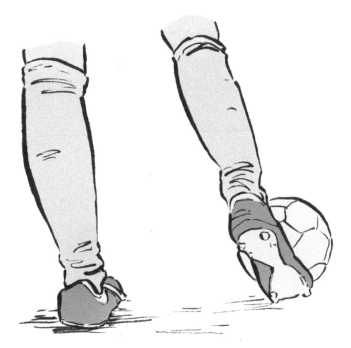

Chipping: Rear View

DRILL

A great way to practice this skill is to play "crossbar challenge" with your friends. It is a fun game, and it will help you practice this technique. In turn, try to hit the bar from outside the 18-yard box. You get 2 points from a stopped ball and 1 point from a moving ball. The first person to 11 points wins!

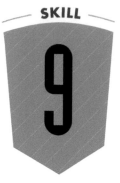

Strike on a Volley

» Passing

Striking the ball on the volley means to hit the ball in the air before it bounces. When you strike the ball on the half volley, you hit the ball after it has bounced once. Both are key techniques to learn, and practice is the key to success. Proper technique is to volley the ball with your hips facing the ball and the target. Focus on finding your balance, getting your eyes on the ball, concentrating on your connection with the ball, and keeping your toe below your ankle at all times.

You can hit the ball on the volley alone against a wall or with a partner about 10 to 15 yards away. Face your partner and hold the ball in both hands at your hips. Let the ball go, strike the ball with your laces, and land on your kicking foot ahead of your plant foot. On contact, lock your ankle joint. As you bring your foot through the ball, keep your toes below your ankle at all times. This will stop the ball from going in the air. Try to keep the ball below chest height.

For the half volley, use the same process. Throw the ball up just above your head, get your feet moving, and keep your eye on the ball. Watch the ball bounce. As the ball starts to drop down for the second bounce, strike through the ball with your laces. Keep your toe below your ankle at all times, and lock your ankle when you hit the ball.

You now have the basics of volleying the ball. Remember to practice accuracy and technique before you build up your power!

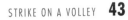

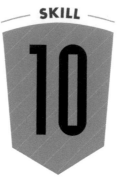

SKILL

10

Take a Penalty

» *Shooting*

Many people believe that penalty taking is luck. These people are usually the ones who miss penalties or play on teams that lose games on penalties. Taking penalties is based on technique, understanding the situation, and confidence. If your technique is good and you understand what you are doing, this gives you the confidence to succeed.

You can't control what the keeper is going to do, and the goals won't move. You control the situation because you control what the ball is going to do. If the keeper guesses right, he or she still won't get to the ball if you hit it well. Remember, the keeper is guessing, and you know where the ball is going.

The two best places to put the ball are low in the corners of the goal or high in the corners of the goal. If the ball goes between the knees and shoulders of the keeper, there is more chance it will be saved. The key to penalties is practice. Place the ball on the spot, decide where it's going if you haven't already, mark out your run the same way a kicker does in the National Football League, breathe, relax, approach the ball, keep your eye on the ball, and hit the target.

Practice this technique as often as possible, with and without a keeper. If you are an accurate penalty taker, you are a valuable asset to your team.

When you make contact with the ball, use the side of your foot or the instep. Place your nonkicking foot slightly ahead of the ball. Lock your ankle. Keep your chest and chin over the ball. Land on your kicking foot, move toward the goal in case the keeper pushes the ball out, and score the rebound.

When taking a penalty, don't change your mind and don't get fancy! Concentrate on the process and not the outcome.

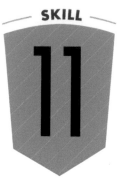

SKILL

11

Shield the Ball

» *Practice with friends*

Shielding the ball is an important skill to learn and a good skill to have so you can keep possession of the ball when you have no other options. You should only shield the ball when you can't turn to face the defender or you have no chance to pass the ball. If this happens, you need to be able to shield the ball until one of the following four things happen:

1. **As you are shielding the ball, the defender tries to come around you to get the ball.** If the defender does this, get away from him or her by getting out the other side.

2. **The defender gets too tight to you and makes contact.** When this happens, use your body to roll off the defender and escape.

3. **A second defender comes and puts pressure on you.** When this happens, if you have your head up, you will see a space that opens up as you become double-teamed.

4. **You get support from a player from your team.** When this happens, you can play the ball to the support player. If you feel really confident, you can use him or her as a decoy and spin away.

To be able to do any of these things, make sure you are in a good position to shield the ball. Get your body between the defender and the ball, and make sure the ball is on the foot farthest away from the defender so he or she can't dangle a leg and get a touch. Then, put the sole of your foot on the ball and use the outside of your foot to move the ball. If your foot is on top of the ball, you are off-balance, and it's harder for you to make your move. Finally, plan your escape and get out of there quickly. If you take more than three or four seconds, you will probably lose the ball.

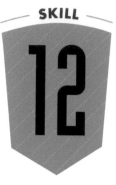

SKILL

12

Juggle the Ball

» *Practice Alone*

Sometimes it's difficult to practice on your own. For many skills you need a partner, but for juggling, all you need is a ball and space to practice. Juggling is a key technique to learn. Every time you make contact with the ball, you are practicing your first touch, which is very important if you want to be a top player.

There are two kinds of ball juggling: straight juggling, where you try to keep the ball off the floor as long as possible and get as many touches as you can, and pattern juggling, where you try to use different surfaces of the foot and different parts of your body in sequence (for example, right foot, left foot, head, thigh, and repeat).

With straight juggling, it's freestyle. Whatever you want, whenever you want! Most of the time, your toe will point up on contact to spin the ball back so you can keep it close and get lots of touches. This will help you in tight spaces when you are surrounded by the other team.

Pattern juggling is a little different because you try to use parts of your body in order. When you practice pattern juggling, challenge yourself and use your weaker foot and less-used parts of your body, such as your chest or thighs. This will help you develop the skill and improve your technique when it comes to controlling the ball in open play.

Juggling the ball is also great for developing balance because most of the time you have one foot off the ground.

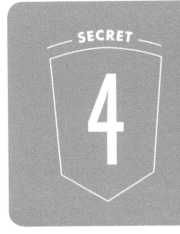

SECRET 4

PICK A ROLE MODEL

Watch players who play in your position on your local team. Copy their movements and learn from their mistakes.

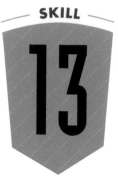

SKILL

13

Play with Both Feet

» Dribbling

Ball manipulation is all about getting touches on the ball and being comfortable with the ball at your feet. Your goal is to try to develop skills with *both* feet. It's challenging to become a two-footed player, but the rewards are great. If you can use both feet, you will be a great asset to your coach and any team on which you play. These activities are similar to juggling because you can run or dribble the ball around or you can set some patterns to follow.

When you start working with the ball, always start with your weaker foot first so you are challenged right from the start. Dribble out to the six-yard line using the inside and outside of your weaker foot, make a turn, and go back to the goal line. Then, go out to the penalty spot, turn, and go back; go out to the top of the 18-yard box and back to the goal line. Repeat these steps with your stronger foot. When you do this exercise, challenge yourself to complete two sets with your weaker foot for every one set with your stronger foot. This will really help you develop your technique. Count your touches and try to increase the number of touches each time. You can also have someone time you and see if you can break your record each day.

Focus on the following: getting your chin up and away from your chest so you can see where you are going, taking small touches so you keep the ball in your safe space and away from defenders, and bending your knees so you can make quick side-to-side movements to beat the defenders.

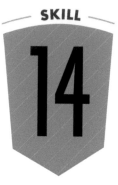

Shoot from Inside the Box

» *Shooting*

Shooting inside the box, or the 18-yard area, is a totally separate technique from shooting from a longer distance. It is more about placement and control than power and pace. Very often, the penalty box is crowded, and it's hard to get a clear sight of the goal. Although this isn't a good situation for you, it's also difficult for the keeper. The keeper will find it hard to see the ball, and it could be deflected. Focus on the following three things when shooting inside the box:

1. Be confident and take a risk. If you don't try a shot, you definitely won't score a goal. The worst thing that can happen is that you miss. The best thing is that you score a goal that helps your team.

2. **Think of it as passing the ball into the goal.** Go for accuracy and a clean contact on your foot instead of trying to blast the ball home.

3. **Keep your feet moving and stay balanced.** If you are falling back or stretching when you make contact with the ball, the chances are good that you won't hit the target.

Once you have these things in place, consider what type of shot you will make and where it should go. Your goal is to hit the target and make the keeper have to save the ball. Shooting over or shooting wide gives the team no chance of a rebound or possible deflection. If possible, try to keep the shot low and below knee height, because that is a difficult place for the keeper to get the ball. If you are inside the frame of the goal when you shoot, just hit the target. However, if you are shooting from a wider position, try to direct your shot across the goal because there are more chances for rebounds and deflections.

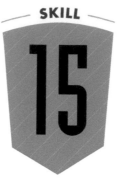

Shoot against the Keeper

» Passing » Shooting

Before you start this exercise, ask yourself, "What can I control in the situation?" You have no control over what the keeper does, and the goal won't move. You only have control over the ball and your own movement, so these things should be your focus when you practice and you are in the game.

Start at the back of the center circle facing the goal. Take a big touch, push the ball 10 to 12 yards out, and sprint after the ball. On your first touch, slow down and push the ball to the left or right. If you are right-footed, go to your right, and if you are left-footed, go to your left. Get your head up and move toward the penalty area. As you approach the penalty area, the ideal place to be is level with the space where the six-yard box is connected to the goal line.

Get your head up, take a breath, and pass the ball into the opposite corner with the inside of your foot. There is no keeper, so you are working on accuracy of the side-foot pass into the far corner of the goal. Repeat this exercise with your opposite foot and on the opposite side of the penalty area.

You should work on this exercise without a keeper a minimum of 30 times on each side before you add the keeper. Your goal is to develop a pattern of movement and breathing that *you* control.

When you add the keeper, be patient with your performance. In a breakaway situation, you have two outcomes: score or don't score! The process of approaching the goal in a controlled manner and hitting the target will eventually lead to success. When you hit your target consistently, you will score goals.

Christine Sinclair

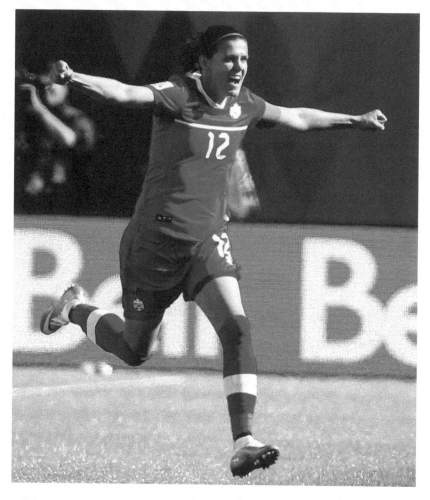

BORN: June 12, 1983 **POSITION:** Forward; attacking midfielder
TEAM: Canadian national team; Portland Thorns FC in
National Women's Soccer League; FC Gold Pride and
Western New York Flash in Women's Professional Soccer

WHEN CHRISTINE SINCLAIR BURST ONTO the world stage at the Fédération Internationale de Football Association U19 Women's Championship, scoring 10 goals and helping Canada earn a silver medal, no one in North America was run down surprised. By then, she had already played in a number of major tournaments for Canada and started her All-American career at the University of Portland.

At Portland, Sinclair led her team to two National Championships in 2002 and 2005. During her college career, she scored 110 goals in 94 games and had 32 assists. Sinclair won championships with FC Gold Pride and Western New York Flash, and she helped Portland Thorns FC win the 2013 Championship. Sinclair helps her team win championships everywhere she plays. Great players make good teams great!

Even though Sinclair is still playing, she will most likely be remembered for a fantastic hat trick in the semi-final of the 2012 London Olympics. There she scored all three goals for Canada in a narrow 4–3 defeat to the United States in what is seen by many as the greatest women's soccer game in history.

What makes Christine Sinclair a superstar? She is not only a great goal scorer, but also a great team player. When Sinclair is double-teamed, she works to create space and chances for her teammates so they can score. When her team is having a tough time, you can always rely on Sinclair to do something to change the game. She holds many goal-scoring records at club and international levels, but her greatest contribution to her team is her great leadership and being a great team player. She is a true superstar.

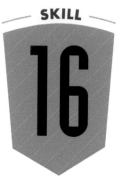

Bend the Ball: Outside

» Passing » Shooting

Using the outside of your foot to bend the ball is one of the hardest skills in the game, but with patience and a lot of practice, you can learn this valuable technique. It is all about getting your feet in the right place, making good contact with the ball, and concentrating on technique rather than power. Once you have the technique in place, you can start to work on power.

Your goal is to get the ball to spin. If you use your *right foot*, it will *spin clockwise*, and if you use your *left foot*, it will *spin counter-clockwise*. Spinning the ball is the key to this skill. Practice this on your own or with a friend who is around 15 to 20 yards away, and start with a ball that is not moving.

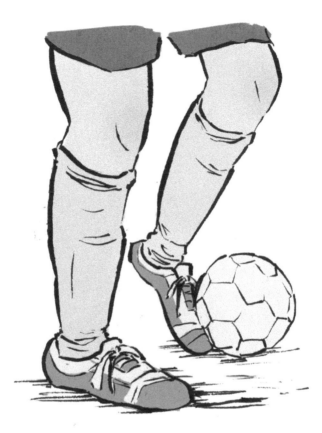

Outside of the Foot

With this skill, place your nonkicking foot at the side of the ball. This time, place yourself a little behind the ball so your kicking foot has room to come through the ball. Take a few steps back and step into the kick like a National Football League kicker. On contact, your toe is pointed down and your heel is up. You are now hitting the ball on the inside, the side nearest to your nonkicking foot. Keep your eye on the ball, look for the spin, and land on your kicking foot ahead of your plant foot. You are using a smaller part of your foot to connect with the ball, so be patient with yourself as you are learning this technique.

SECRET

5

WATCH LIVE GAMES

When you watch a live game, you can really see what is happening all over the field, and it will make you a better player. Check out your local team.

Head the Ball

» Passing » Shooting

Heading the ball is a big part of being a soccer player. If you can't head the ball, it will be harder to play at the highest level you desire. Heading the ball can also be very dangerous if you don't learn to do it correctly. Heading the ball correctly will help you become a better player. However, more important than becoming a good soccer player is being a safe and healthy soccer player.

You'll want to consider the following:

- You don't have to head every ball 30 yards, but you do have to head every ball with the correct technique.

- You head the ball; the ball doesn't hit your head.

When you are learning to head the ball, the best person to coach you is probably yourself. Throw the ball in the air just above your head, and practice heading the ball back up and catching it. Use the bony part of your forehead just above your nose and two-thirds of the way up your forehead. If you head the ball on the top part of your head, it will hurt and can be dangerous. As you become comfortable with the technique, you can start to head a ball that is thrown to you from 5 to 10 yards and then 10 to 15 yards.

When you head the ball defensively in a game, head the ball up and away. If you are attacking and trying to score, head the ball down and at the goal.

Heading the ball is a complex skill. Your coach will be able to help you develop your technique during practice, but if you also practice by yourself, you help your coach, while becoming a better player. Remember, safety and correct technique are the key to success.

STRATEGIES

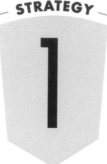

Learn by Watching

» *Defending*

There is nothing better than practice to help you improve your game. It's also good for you to watch soccer so you can see how the players move and what they do when they are away from the ball. When games are shown on television, the camera often focuses on the ball because people watching at home want to see what happens with the ball and see all of the action.

Have you ever wondered why coaches of professional teams go to watch other teams play? After all, they could sit at home and watch the game like everyone else. They go to watch games so they can see the things you can't see on television. For example, they want to see how a team is organized when they are going forward, where players go after they pass the ball, and what the movement of the strikers is like when the ball is in midfield. As a player learning the game, there are many things you can pick up from watching your local major league soccer or college team play.

When you go to the game, take a notepad so you can jot down notes about what is happening. It can be hard to remember everything without taking notes. There are several things you may want to watch during the game that will help you better understand how top-level players and teams play soccer. It's best to watch players who play the same position as you, so you can learn some of their tricks and see how they move.

If you are a striker or player in a wide position, pay close attention to what the players do when their team doesn't have the ball. What positions do they take up? What are their body positions? Are they flat-footed and resting, or are they on their toes and ready to move? The key moment to watch them is when their team wins the ball back. Look for their movement patterns in transition, and see what you can use in your game.

If you are watching defenders, take a close look at them when their team starts to build up an attack. What positions do they take up? Do they look to join the attack, or do they stay back? How do they prepare for the next time the team has to defend? How close are they to the player they are marking when the ball is far away? How do they close spaces down when the ball comes toward them? If you are a defender, the answers to these questions will make you a better player.

If you are a midfielder, watch the movement of the players who play in midfield. How often do they get the ball? What do they do with it when they have it? How often do they win the ball back, and how often do they give possession away? Watching an expert play in your position is a great way to become a better player.

In addition to watching these players, spend 15 to 20 minutes focusing on how the team plays as a group. How do they attack? Do they use long passes or short buildup play? Do they attack through the middle of the field or use the wings of the field? What do they do as a group when they lose the ball? Do they drop back to their own goal and "park the bus," or do they try to pressure the ball and win it back quickly?

Watching games will help you develop as a player, and it will also impress your coach.

Remember and Predict Patterns

» *Passing*

When you watch a game of soccer, it can be very difficult to see what is really happening and it can seem very confusing. As you get older, the games you play will become a little more organized. Right now, you and your teammates are still learning to play the game, so the games may still feel like a random series of events happening all over the field. It is important to learn to recognize patterns in the game and be able to anticipate what is coming next.

Let's compare a game of soccer to your favorite movie or story. If you see a movie on the weekend and then see that same movie the following weekend, you will see exactly the same thing. There will be a start to the movie where you are introduced to the characters, a middle part of the movie where the plot thickens, and at the end of the movie, the good guys win and the credits roll. Each second of the movie has 24 frames, and these frames will be in exactly the same order each time you watch this movie the rest of your life. It's the same with a book. You start at the first page and keep going until you run out of pages.

Think about a game of soccer like this: The only thing that is the same in any game of soccer is the start to the "movie" and the end of the movie. The referee blows the whistle to start the game, and the referee blows the whistle to signal the end. There is a plot to the game: there are goal kicks, free kicks, corners, throw-ins, fouls, offside decisions, goals, passes given away, good passes to teammates, and many other little actions or events. The difference between a game of soccer and a movie or a book is that the pages of soccer games *never* happen in the same order. In almost all of our games, all of the pages are there, just in a *different* order. Understanding this idea is the key to developing your skills in recognizing patterns in play and developing the skill of anticipation.

If a coach was asked to describe one skill present in all of the world's best soccer players, it would most likely be that "they always know where the ball is going to be before anyone else." The best players don't *really* know where the ball is going, but they "feel" where the ball is going and they do this using a skill called pattern recognition. This means that they remember seeing something happen in a game or practice, and they make a decision on where to go or what to do based on their memory of what happened before. Even the world's best soccer players don't get everything right. But when you do recognize a pattern and react to it correctly in a game, everyone will see!

DRILL

A good way to help you develop the skill of pattern recognition is to play "rock, paper, scissors" with your friends. Pay attention to their moves and see if you can predict what they will do next.

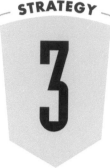

STRATEGY

3

Be Aware of Your Space

» *Running*

Your goal is to find space as it opens up and be available to receive a pass. Soccer fields are up to 9,600 square yards, but finding space can sometimes be very difficult. Against better players and better teams, it becomes even harder. You will need to learn where you can find space and, more importantly, where can you find space that hurts the opposition. The key to finding space is to be aware of the area around you. Your coach may call this "spatial awareness."

How do you develop spatial awareness? The most important thing to do is to keep "sneaking a peek" over your shoulder so you get a picture of the whole field and start to understand where the spaces are. You will learn many times by reading this book that, when you have an understanding of where players are, where they came from, and where they are going, it will help you stand out from the crowd.

There is a lot of space on the field. Most players focus on the ball and don't pay attention to what is happening away from the ball, which is how you look for space. To help your team, any space is a good space as long as you are supporting the ball carrier. However, it is important to know that there is good space, better space, and the best space.

Finding space behind the ball is good. This means finding space closer to your team's goal than the ball. This allows you to see what is happening down the field, but the team is moving backward, so you need to be ready to play quickly. Pressure will be coming!

If the ball is in the center of the field, finding space on the wings is better because it will move the other team's defenders across the field. When you have the ball wide on either side of the field, your options are limited because you can go only up, down, or inside. The best space to find, although the hardest space to find, is space ahead of the ball. This means space closer to the opponent's goal than the ball. This is where you have to work hard to get free and your ability to be spatially aware is very important.

Make sure you are constantly checking where the ball is. Defenders will be moving toward the ball, so you need to see where they are coming from and check to see if the space stays open or is closed by another defender.

Defenders most likely won't be marking you if you start your run from behind the ball, because you don't pose a threat to them. If you can make a run past the ball into space, it makes you a real asset to your team. If you start your run in the middle of the field and run to the line, you can get stuck there and become easy to mark. It is better to start a run from the outside and come inside. That way, even if you don't get the ball, it's easier to make another run to find space from that position.

Your ability to be spatially aware and sneak a peek over your shoulder will improve your ability to know where space will appear.

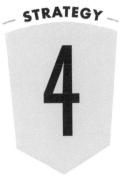

4

Receive a Pass

» *Practice with friends*

When you are learning to play soccer, it's difficult to take your eyes off the ball, because you are not always sure where the ball is, even when it is at your feet. Over time, this will change as you become a more experienced player. When you develop the skill of getting your head up as the ball comes to you and learn how to "open up" your body to receive a pass, it will really help you in the game.

When you receive a pass from a teammate with your hips and feet facing him or her, this is a closed position because you can only pass the ball back to your teammate. When you open your body up, you move your feet as the ball comes to you, so when you receive the pass, you see the space to which you want to pass or move into with the ball. This sounds straightforward, but many players are not able to easily master this skill. If you do, you will be a great asset to your team.

These simple movements will greatly improve your soccer game. As you get more comfortable with this skill, you will notice that, as you open up your body, your head turns so you can see the space that was behind you. You are now automatically sneaking a peek, which gives you more information and lets you make better decisions about what to do next. As you start to open up your body, you will notice that sometimes you don't have to control the ball and you can use the weight of the pass to keep moving in the direction you want to go.

DRILL

The best way to learn this movement is to practice with your friends. Start 10 yards apart and make simple passes to one another. Have your feet face the ball. As the ball comes to you, move your left foot behind you so that your shoulder is facing the passer. Let the ball run past your right foot, and use your left foot to control the ball. Now, repeat this action, but move your right foot back, let the ball run past your left foot, and receive the ball on your right foot.

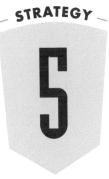

Stay Onside

» *Running*

One of the most controversial moments in the game for players, coaches and fans is when a goal is called back for being offside.

The offside rule seems to change a lot, and it is the source of many arguments among fans. Coaches also argue with officials about the offside rule, but it is pointless because once you are given offside, you are offside. The offside rule may appear to change, but to beat the rule, when the ball is passed forward, there has to be two players from the other team, including the keeper, between you and the opponent's goal. It becomes a little more difficult when players start to move around.

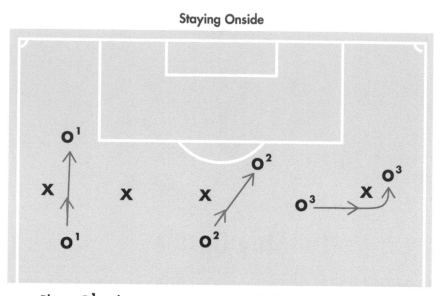

Player **O^1** makes a poor run in a straight line.
Player **O^2** makes a better diagonal run.
Player **O^3** makes the best run, with a hook turn at the end.

How do you stay onside? Be aware of where your opponent's back line is on the field, get your chin off your chest, keep looking to see where they are, and adjust your movement accordingly. Staying onside in wide positions can be a little easier. If you open your body up to the field and get your toes and hips pointing to the center of the field, you should be able to see across the back line and stay onside as play is developing. It becomes a little more challenging in the center of the field because you have to keep turning your head to check the position of the back line. Being aware of your surroundings will make you a better player, so take the chance to play in the center whenever you can. Remember that if you get caught offside, it's not the end of the world. It's a learning opportunity, and learning opportunities are priceless.

The next part of staying onside is based on your movement into space to receive the ball. If you make a run up the field in a straight line, you will likely be caught offside if the pass you want is delayed. If you make a run into an offside position and don't get the ball, try to get back onside as quickly as possible so you can help your team. The best type of run to make is a horizontal run across the field in front of the defense with a hook turn just after the pass is made, which will keep you onside. Just as good is a diagonal run across the defender. Start this run from a position two or three steps onside and make sure you can see the pass so you can time your break into open space.

The last piece of the puzzle is what to do when you get "caught" offside. Think of beating the offside trap as a game of cat and mouse. Sometimes you get caught when you were onside, and sometimes you will get away with being offside. It's how you react to the official's decision that makes the difference. Soccer is a game of mistakes and how you react to those mistakes. If you get caught offside and complain, chances are good that you won't get the benefit of the doubt on the next close call. If you accept the official's decision, you will be going through on a breakaway sooner rather than later.

6

What to Do in Wide Positions

» *Defending* » *Passing* » *Running*

One of the most demanding positions to play is the wide position in midfield. This position also includes the wide striker if your team plays with three players up front. If you don't play smart, you will run out of steam very quickly!

When your team is defending, everyone wants you to get back. When your team has the ball, everyone is shouting for you to get forward. When you're running up and down the field to help everyone, you're bound to get tired, and when you get tired, it is easy for you to get sloppy with your technique and make poor decisions. What can you do to become an effective wide midfielder and help your team?

Talk with your coach before games and at practices so you know what he or she wants you to do. If your coach wants you to join the attack, ask how far you should drop down the field when your team is defending. This will help you take up a good position for when your team wins the ball. However, your coach might want you to play a more defensive role. Then you need to ask how far up the field you should go when your team is attacking and what your position should be to support players on the ball. The most important question to ask your coach is, "Where is my starting position when we win the ball?" This will help you figure out where to be and how much of the field you have to cover in the game. When you get this information, you have a better chance of helping the team.

If you are a wide midfielder, it's also very important when you get the ball that your first touch to control it is into a safe space so you can secure the ball and keep possession. Make sure you open your body up so when you receive the ball, you can see the whole field from the wide position. As you have learned, when you open up your body, you have a better view of the field and a better chance of making a good decision. If you make a pass, you need to get in a position to either support the pass or make a run to create space. As you play soccer more, this will become easier. There isn't a right or wrong in this situation. It is just you making a decision based on what you see. Don't be afraid to make a decision. That is what your coach wants you to do.

When your team doesn't have the ball and is defending, the first question to ask yourself is, "Am I in the right spot to help my team?" If the answer is "yes," that's great. If the answer is "no," can you get to that spot as soon as possible? When you are defending, the easiest thing to do is to drop all the way down and get closer to your goal. Think about this: If you get too close to the full back, you help the other team because you opened up a space the opposing players can fill and you won't be able to get up the field to support your team's next attack.

Playing in wide positions can be difficult, but it will become easier as you get more experience. Make communication with your coach a priority. For a soccer team to be successful, it needs players who can play wide positions well.

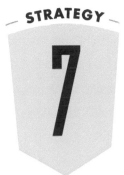

Get Behind the Ball

» *Defending*

When your team loses possession of the ball, the first thing you should do is get into a position to help your team defend. If your team has the ball for half of the game and you don't help them defend, this means you are playing only 50 percent of the game. Think of it like this: If you answered only half of the questions on a test at school, you would still receive a grade of "F" even if you answered them all correctly. There is no room for a failing grade on your team, either.

When your team loses the ball, the first question to ask yourself is, "Am I in the right place to help my team defend?" If the answer is "no," you need to get to that place as quickly as possible. As a rule, when your team loses the ball, you want to try to recover behind the ball. This means you are closer to your own goal than the ball. If you can get between the ball and your own goal, it is a good position to be in because the ball has to go past you in order for the other team to have a chance to score. This may sound like common sense, but many players don't pay attention to the game; instead they stand and watch the other team attack. Your coach will appreciate you trying to recover behind the ball because it shows you are a team player. Even if you are playing in a forward position, you should still make the effort to get back and help your midfielders. The best players in the world, such as the superstars mentioned in this book, all work hard for their teams.

Let's look at how you recover to a position behind the ball and help your team. As soon as your team loses the ball, move back down the field so you can get into a defensive position. From your position on the field, imagine a line to the center of your team's goal. This is your recovery line and the quickest route to a spot behind the ball. Sometimes just making a move back toward your own goal will disrupt the other team's plans and help your team. If you are in a wide position, try to get "inside of the ball" as soon as possible. This means you are closer to the center of the field than the ball. By taking up a position in the center of the field, you help your team keep the ball on one side, making it easier to defend.

As you get closer to the ball, you need to decide whether to try to get the ball or get into a covering position and help the first defender. If there is no one from your team close to the ball carrier, you will need to pressure the ball. Remember, don't try to tackle from behind, because that will be a foul. Get back behind the ball and put some pressure on the ball. If someone from your team is in position to defend, get close to that player and offer support to help him or her win the ball back.

To recap, get on the recovery line as soon as you can. Try to get inside of the ball and help fill the middle of the field. Pressure the ball if no one is around it, and offer support if your teammate is defending the ball.

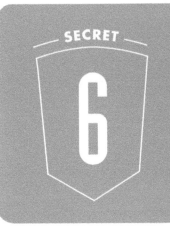

SECRET

6

STAY IN SHAPE

Your coach isn't a fitness trainer. Take responsibility for your own fitness level and don't fall behind. Be the fittest player on the team.

Mia Hamm

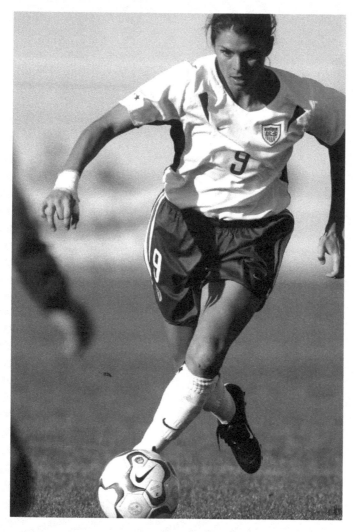

BORN: March 17, 1972 **POSITION:** Forward
TEAM: US women's national soccer team

WOMEN'S SOCCER IS VERY POPULAR around the world and especially in the United States. One of the most influential players in the history of the sport is Mia Hamm. Hamm is 5 feet and 5 inches tall, but when she played soccer, she was the biggest player on the field.

When playing, Hamm was a predator and the most dangerous forward around. Her movement to create space for herself was fantastic, and many of her teammates were able to score goals because of the space she created for them.

Hamm played 275 games for the US women's national soccer team and scored 158 goals, which is a great strike rate. She was also a key member of the 1991 and 1999 US Women's World Cup teams. Along with her two World Cup winners' medals, she won two Olympic gold medals in 1996 and 2004. Shortly after the 2004 Olympics, she retired from playing soccer. In her whole college soccer career at the University of North Carolina, Hamm's team lost only one game when she was playing. Great players make good teams great, and Hamm made every team she played for great.

Mia Hamm's contribution to the game of soccer as a player is huge, but her work away from the field has been equally important. Mia became the face of women's soccer and a role model for young players to follow. When Mia Hamm first started playing soccer, women's soccer was a sport that didn't generate a lot of interest. When she retired in 2004, women's soccer had become an important sport watched by millions around the world. Mia Hamm certainly helped that happen and became one of the sport's first superstars.

8

Take a Throw-In

» *Passing*

In each game, on average, there are about 45 throw-ins. If you assume your team will get half of them, your team has between 20 and 23 chances to keep the ball each game after the other team has kicked the ball out. This means throw-ins are a very important part of a soccer game. If your team learns to keep the ball after a throw-in, you will increase the amount of time you have the ball in the game. Remember, having the ball more than the other team doesn't mean you will win the game. However, if the other team has less time with the ball to create scoring opportunities, then your team will become harder to beat!

There are important things to know about throw-ins when your team has the ball. It is also good to know what you can do as an individual player to help your team in two specific situations.

When you are taking the throw-in, don't rush and end up making a foul throw. Make sure that you do the following:

- Face the field of play.

- Have part of each foot either on the touchline or on the ground behind the touchline.

- Use both hands.

- Throw the ball from behind and over your head.

When you throw the ball to a player on your team, make sure that he or she can control it with one touch, or even better, he or she can move the ball to the next player, which could be you with one touch. Look at this as a pass with your hands. The best pass is to a player's feet or maybe even to the head so it can be directed to another teammate. Throwing it at the face, shoulders, chest, or waist won't help. If you do this, it's possible your teammate will lose possession of the ball. As with passing, think about your teammate and give that person the best chance to succeed. Remember, after you throw the ball, move to a position of support.

Receive a Throw-In

» *Defending* » *Passing*

To keep possession when you receive a throw-in, it is most important that your first touch is consistent and reliable. This is something you should take responsibility for and practice as often as possible.

The second thing to think about is the timing of your movement into the space to receive the throw-in. If you get there too early, you will attract another defender and bring more players around the ball. This makes it harder for the player throwing the ball. When this happens, everyone moves closer to the ball, and there is a good chance possession will be lost. If you get there too late, the ball also is lost. This takes time to learn, so be patient with yourself.

The last thing to think about is what part of your body you will use to connect with the ball. If you are trying to play one-touch, it has to be either your foot or your head to give you the best chance to succeed. Your focus is on keeping possession of the ball, so keep things as simple as possible.

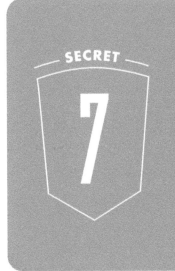

WEAR THE PROPER SHOES AND CLOTHING

Make sure you have the proper footwear for the playing conditions. If you have trouble moving around because of your clothes, you won't be a help to your team.

10

Know Common Patterns

» *Defending* » *Passing*

Now that you have a basic understanding of pattern recognition and how it can help you become a better player, let's look at cues that help you predict what might happen next and how you can react to them.

There are patterns to look for when your team is defending. Your focus now is on trying to stop the other team from doing things that help them score.

On a goal kick, if the *center backs split apart*, this could be a cue for their center midfielder to drop down and get the ball at his or her feet so he or she can play from the back. If you see this happen, try to get close enough to the player to stop him or her from receiving the ball. This will force the player to kick the ball out wide to a defender who may not be as good with the ball.

When your team is *defending a corner*, if the other team sends two people over to take the corner, they are most likely trying to take a short corner. To stop this from happening, go out to the corner flag with another defender to make it a 2-vs.-2 situation. This will force the other team to do something different.

If the team you are playing against likes to *pass the ball around their back four and build up slowly*, try to take up a position that cuts out a pass between the center backs. This will help the rest of your team because you can keep the other team on one side of the field and take their space away.

When you are *defending a throw-in*, if the player you are marking makes a run toward the player throwing the ball and gets too close, don't follow that player all the way. If you do, you open up a space behind yourself that the ball can be thrown into. Always be aware of the space you are leaving.

If you are *playing the back line*, try to focus on the hips of the ball carrier. If they open up, a long ball may be coming. Drop back to increase your chances of getting to the ball first.

There are also some things you can look for *when your team has the ball*. If you play in midfield, look for your strikers to make a move toward the ball to receive a pass. If you see this happening, make a run into the space they just left. You will be unmarked and most likely in on the goal.

If you are *taking a free kick* and you want to score, try to look at the keeper's legs to see if they are off-balanced or his or her weight is loaded to one side. If so, this means the keeper will have trouble moving to that side. There is your scoring opportunity! This works with penalties, as well.

Avoid running to the ball if your team is attacking and in the penalty area with the ball. Look for a space on the far post just outside the six-yard box instead. All the defenders will rush to the ball, and you will have space to yourself if you get to it.

Pattern recognition is a skill that you can learn by watching games and playing games, and when you learn it, you will be a much better player. Be patient and trust your instincts.

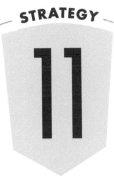

11

Keep the Ball or Pass It?

» Passing » Running » Dribbling

When you get the ball, you have two choices of what to do next. You can keep the ball yourself by running or dribbling with it, or you can make a pass to a teammate directly to his or her feet or to an open space for him or her to run into. It is important to know cues or triggers to look for so you can make the best decision.

If you receive the ball and there is a defender close to you, try to look past the defender to see if there is space there for you to attack. If there is, dribble toward the defender and go for the space behind that player. Remember to keep the ball close to your feet to draw the defender to you, and then explode past him or her into the open space.

If you receive the ball and you have a defender 5 to 10 yards away, move toward the defender and draw him or her to the ball. This will create space for your teammates and give you room to pass. If you get the ball and you have some open space in front of you, your coach will most likely encourage you to run with the ball into the open space and attack your opponent's back line. This will cause the other team lots of problems, and, at some point, someone will have to challenge you. If you are moving more quickly than the challenger and you have the ball under control, you will be able to move past the person easily and draw more of their teammates to the ball. This will create more space for your teammates.

Finally, if you receive the ball and are isolated from the other team, you will have to work hard to keep the ball, and you may have to shield it until support arrives.

When passing the ball, think about why you pass the ball. You pass the ball to move it, but you also can move the ball by dribbling and running with it. However, passing the ball is the quickest way to move the ball.

You also only want to pass the ball to someone who is in a better position than you. Sometimes the ball is passed to players who are marked, which puts them in trouble and at risk of losing the ball. This can be called a "trouble pass" because the player receiving the ball is in trouble and now needs help.

You should pass the ball when you see a player who is unmarked higher up or closer to your opponent's goal than you are. This helps the team, and is a called a "positive pass," meaning that, after the pass, your team is in a better position either higher up the field or the player on the ball has more space, even if the pass has gone backward (it can't always go forward).

The last thing to look at is the distance of your pass. A player who is unmarked 40 yards away might be marked tightly by the time your pass lands at his or her feet. So, what you thought was a positive pass has turned into a trouble pass because the defenders have moved to the ball or anticipated your pass.

When you're playing in a game, keep track of the number of positive passes you make and try to increase the number in each game.

Lionel Messi

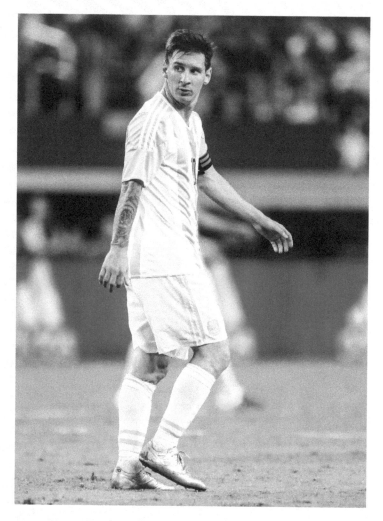

BORN: June 24, 1987 **POSITION:** Forward
TEAM: Barcelona; Argentina national soccer team

TWO WORDS YOU HEAR TOGETHER a lot are "Messi" and "goal." It seems like all Lionel Messi does is score goals for Barcelona and Argentina, but there is so much more to know about Messi.

When he was very young, he was diagnosed with a medical condition that prevented him from growing normally, and he had to receive treatment to help him grow.

He left Argentina with his father to join the Barcelona Soccer Academy when he was just 11 years old. During his time with the Barcelona academy, he won every major club medal and played a key role in Barcelona's dominance of Spain and Europe. He has also represented his country more than 100 times and continues to be a big threat in international football.

Messi has many great talents. He is a great goal scorer, and many opponents and managers have said that when he is playing well, he is virtually unstoppable. His low center of gravity helps him turn quickly to create goal-scoring chances in the box and turn away from defenders in the open field. When Messi receives the ball in open play, his speed and footwork are outstanding, and this is why he is such a formidable player. He is very strong on the ball, and it's almost impossible for defenders to push him out of the way. His acceleration away from defenders creates spaces in other areas of the field for his teammates, and in this way, he also plays a part in assisting with goals.

Lionel Messi is a great team player. He works just as hard when he doesn't have the ball to help his team win the ball back. His work ethic and fantastic skills make him possibly the greatest soccer player of all time.

12

Get Past the Other Team

» *Passing*

How can you get the ball to the goal and create a scoring chance for your team? You can go over, around, or through your opponent. The trick is not only picking the easiest and quickest route to the goal but also having a backup plan if one is needed.

Your first choice is to *go over* your opponent with a through-ball from the midfield area, a long ball from the defenders, or a long ball directly from the keeper with a goal kick or kick from their hands. There are fewer touches involved in this type of move, but at the same time, you can't just kick the ball down the field and hope that it works. That's not soccer! Make controlled passes

Playing Through, Over, and Around

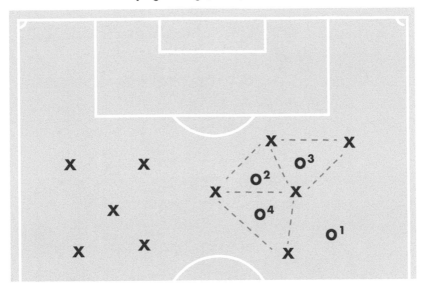

Here the defending team is in a lower block, and spread out. In this case we must play through them by breaking lines and living in the triangle. O^1 has the option to pass to O^2, O^3, or O^4.

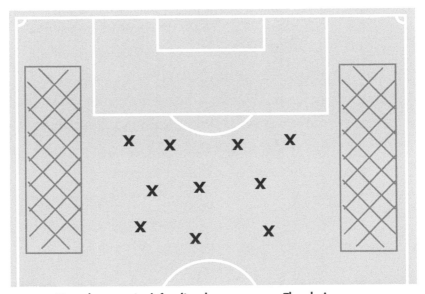

Here the team is defending low + narrow. The choice here is to go around in the shaded areas.

over your opponent into an open space for your team's players to move into. To go over the other team, you need to have space into which you play the ball. If the other team's back line is high up around the halfway line or at the back of the center circle, you will have enough room to attack. If they are playing deep in their half and the back line is down by their penalty area, you can't go over them because there isn't enough space. In this case, you have to find another way.

If the defending team is down low with the back line *around* the edge of the penalty area, look at how they are positioned across the field. This will help you decide how to attack. If their players who are positioned wide are inside of the 18-yard box, this will allow you to attack them around the outside. You will need to get the ball out wide as quickly as possible, and try to get to the goal line and get some crosses in. Quick, accurate passes to the feet of the players who are positioned wide are good. A pass just ahead of them is better so they can run into the space and make the cross. You can also go around the other team if there is some space behind the players. Try to be unpredictable in your play and do different things.

If the other team is low down and evenly spread across the field, go *through* them. This requires a lot of skill and patience, but playing through to the goal makes your team a formidable opponent. Playing through the other team is

Playing Through, Over, and Around

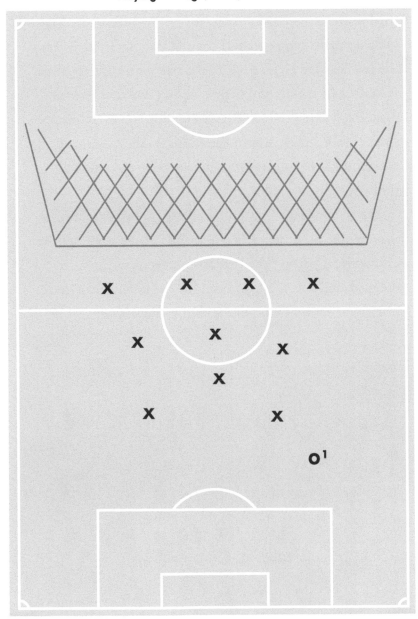

Here the defending team is high up so **O¹** can play the ball over them into the shaded area.

hard because there is no room for error. Your passes have to be accurate and at a good pace so the player receiving the pass has the chance to get the ball with time to spare. A "soft" pass means you will be closed down quickly and most likely lose the ball. Pass accurately, move and create space, sneak a peek, live in the triangles the other team creates, and open up your body to receive the ball—all skills that are covered in this book.

When you learn how and when to go over, around, or through the other team, it will make you a smarter player. Of course, if you get the ball at your feet, you are facing the goal, and you think you can hit the target, then go for it! Remember, you miss every shot you don't take.

PREPARE FOR PRACTICE

Lay out all your equipment before practice so you don't forget anything. Think about what happened in the last practice and how you can be ready for this practice.

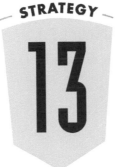

STRATEGY

13

Beat a Player without Touching the Ball

» Passing » Running » Dribbling

The next progression in developing this skill is to beat a player with your movement without touching the ball. In this exercise, instead of stepping back, you move toward the ball. As the pass is made, step toward the ball with your right foot and point your shoulder at the passer. As the ball rolls to you, put your weight on your right foot. As the ball goes past your right foot, push off and let the ball go past you and onto your left foot. Now, repeat the exercise on the other side of your body. Step toward the ball with your left foot, point your shoulder at the passer, and put your weight on your left foot. As the ball rolls past your left foot, push off and let the ball go past you and onto your right foot.

Practice this skill with slow movements, so you understand the timing and the pattern of movement. As you become more comfortable, speed up your movements. Be patient with yourself. This is a very important skill that helps you beat a player without actually touching the ball.

SECRET

9

REHYDRATE AFTER THE GAME

Start drinking as soon as the game ends. Choose sports drinks that help your body replace the electrolytes and carbohydrates you used up during the game.

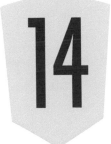

STRATEGY
14

Choose the Right Pass

» *Passing*

Possession of the ball is important, but possession on its own won't win the game. Scoring goals wins the game. Possession is important because if you have the ball, then your opponent can't score!

There are several things to think about when you have the ball at your feet, and there are different types of passes you can make to your teammates. It is also important to know when, where, and why you might take a risk with a pass.

Let's look at two different types of passes: A directional pass is in the direction of the goal that you are attacking. A *possession pass* is a pass that is either horizontal across the field or to a player on your team who is behind the ball. You make a possession pass when you are unable to move forward but need to keep possession of the ball to continue to attack.

Before you make a directional pass, there are several things to consider.

- **How far away is my teammate, and can I get the ball to him or her?** If you can't get the ball to your teammate with a crisp pass, there is a good chance that when it arrives, your teammate will be closely marked and under pressure. It's important to know what your range of passing is with your side-foot pass, mid-range pass, and long-range pass, so you can make the best decision before you pass. These techniques will be covered later in the book.

- **Is the player you are passing to in a better spot than you?** If your teammate is closely marked or isolated from the rest of the team, it's probably not a good idea to pass the ball to him or her. You should only pass the ball to someone who is in a better position than you. If the pass you want to make doesn't help your team, then you are probably making the wrong pass.

If you can't go forward with a pass, it's time to do a possession pass so your team can keep the ball and look for other chances to score. Before you make a possession pass, there are a couple of things to consider.

- **Are you close enough to support the player with the ball when you make the pass?** If so, this type of pass is a good option because there is a good chance you will help your team keep possession of the ball.

- **What options does your teammate have when he or she receives the ball?** If you are passing the ball to a teammate in a central position, the player will most likely be able to go to the left or right when receiving the ball from you. This is much better than passing to someone closer to the touchline, because that player can only come back inside the field.

Whether you make a directional pass or possession pass, think about the player receiving the ball and do your best to help him or her with your pass. The pass needs to be accurate and at a pace that allows your teammate to control the ball, if needed, or play a one-touch pass, if possible. If your pass is too hard or too soft, it could put your teammate in a tough position.

Don't be frightened to take a risk with a pass—be aware of where you are on the field. As a rule, it is best not to take risks with passes in your own defending third, because you don't want to give the ball away in that area. As you move higher up the field, you can take more risks. When you are in your attacking third, you will need to take risks with passes and shots to create scoring chances.

SECRET

10

EAT TO SUCCEED

Carbohydrates act as fuel for your body. Eating a banana an hour before the game will give you a carbohydrate boost and fill your gas tank.

15

Help the Player on the Ball

» Passing

When your team has the ball, supporting the player with the ball is the most important thing you can do. Your coach might use the terms "first attacker" for the player with the ball, "second attacker" for the player nearest to the ball carrier, and "third attacker" for everyone else on the team. Let's look at the best positions you can take so if you get the ball, you can keep the ball and make the next pass.

The best type of supporting position is when you face the player with the ball, so the player can make a pass to someone he or she easily sees. You might have to work a little harder to get into this space, but your job is to help

Helping the Player on the Ball

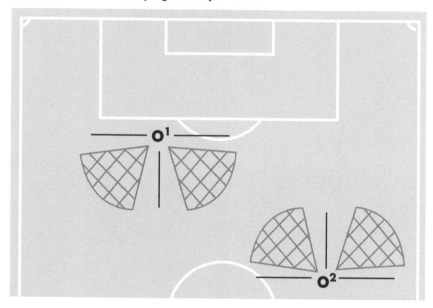

For **O**[1] the shaded areas are good supporting positions as **O**[1] has their back to the goal. For **O**[2] the shaded areas are good supporting positions as **O**[2] is facing the goal. *Don't be in a horizontal or vertical position to the ball.*

the ball carrier. If you call for a pass and the player with the ball can't see you, the player will have to guess where you are. If his or her guess is wrong, your team will have to get the ball back!

Think about where you will be when you call for the ball. Always look for a supporting position that is away from a straight line so you are supporting the ball carrier on an angle. If your supporting position is in a straight line directly behind the ball carrier, the defending team doesn't have to move across the field to deal with your attacking position, and you want to make them move around as much as possible. If you offer support in a straight line across the field, it will be a risky pass. If it gets intercepted, both you and your teammate are out of the defensive position and on the wrong side of the ball because your team is now defending. If you offer support ahead of the ball in a straight line, this can be a problem for you if you get the pass. When you receive a straight pass from a player who is down the field, it is easy for the defender to get in a good, tight position because he or she is able to see you and the ball as it comes to you.

If you take up a position on an angle to the ball carrier as the ball comes to you, opening up your body will help you find a space to beat the defender as he or she close in on you. As you play more and practice with your team, you will see that a supporting position on an angle is the best spot for you.

You will also want to think about the distance between you and the player you want to support. If you are too far away, the pass may be intercepted before you get a chance to receive the ball. If you get too close, you may bring an extra defender with you and make it harder for the player with the ball. Of course, by bringing another player closer to the ball, you will open up a space somewhere else. There is no right or wrong distance. It is trial and error, and the more times you try different things, the more quickly you will learn.

The last thing to consider is if you can get to the best position. If you are too far away, try to anticipate the next pass and get into a position to support that player. Always try to think one pass ahead.

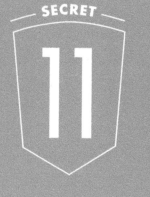

SECRET **BE A TEAM PLAYER**

For example, bring along an extra water bottle to games and practices. Someone usually forgets his or her drink. Without being hydrated, players can't help their team.

16

Help Your Team Defend

» *Defending*

You should always play a part in winning the ball back regardless of what your position may be. When you are not the player who is closest to the ball, you still have a role in helping your team defend. The defender who is closest to the ball is always called the "first defender." The first defender's job is to put the ball carrier under pressure and delay the attack. If you find yourself close to the first defender, you are the "second defender," or covering defender. Your job is to get in a position to cover the first defender and offer support. As you develop as a player, you will learn to communicate with the first defender to help your team win the ball back.

Your positioning is very important in order to help your teammates defend. Find a position that isn't too close to the ball but not too far away. If you get too close to the ball, you will have opened up a space somewhere else, and if you are playing a good team, the player with the ball will see this and probably pass to an open player or an open space. At the same time, if you get too close, you might confuse the first defender, and any miscommunication will let the player on the ball get free. If you are too far away, you are not offering support to the first defender, leaving him or her isolated and at risk of getting beaten in a 1-vs.-1 situation.

Where is the right position? It's difficult to show a diagram of the right position to be in, because the ball and players are always moving. It's better for you to know what your responsibilities are so, over time, you will figure out the best position to be in as a supporting defender.

Take up a position behind the first defender and position your body so you can see the ball carrier, your defending partner, and the space the attacking team is trying to get to. Now, get close enough to your partner so if he or she decides to tackle the ball, you are close enough to win the ball if your partner doesn't succeed. At the same time, be far enough away so you can get in a position to intercept any pass or at least put pressure on the player who receives the pass. If this happens, you become the first defender, and you know what is involved in that role.

This may sound quite complicated, but the more games you play, the better you will become. Be patient and set realistic goals. You have lots of time to learn to play soccer, and your coach is there to help you. When you watch soccer, whether at a live game or on television, pay attention to the defending team. Try to pick out the first defender and covering defender, and watch how they move and readjust their positions as the ball moves.

SECRET

12

PREPARE FOR PRACTICE

What do you want to achieve this coming season? Set goals you can measure such as, "This season, I will practice my short-passing accuracy until I miss only half as many short passes as I missed last year."

Alex Morgan

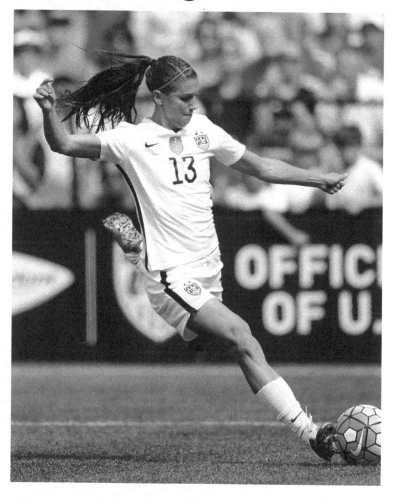

BORN: July 2, 1989 **POSITION:** Forward
TEAM: US women's national soccer team;
Orlando Pride, Western New York Flash,
Seattle Sounders, Portland Thorns FC

ONE OF THE MOST INTERESTING things about Alex Morgan, one of soccer's youngest and brightest superstars, is that as a child she was a multi-sport athlete and didn't start playing club soccer until the age of 14. Within three years she was called up to play with the US women's national soccer team. She was just 17 years old.

In college at UC Berkeley, Alex played for the California Golden Bears and scored an impressive 45 goals. Even though she graduated a year early, she still ranks third in all-time scoring for the Bears. In club soccer, she was the first overall pick for the Western New York Flash in the 2011 Women's Professional Soccer draft. She then moved to the Seattle Sounders for the 2012 season, and later played with the Portland Thorns FC where she helped win the National Women's Soccer League Championship in 2015.

Her greatest achievements and performances have come at the very highest level with the US women's national soccer team. In 2012 she became an Olympic gold medalist and was named the US Women's Player of the Year. In 2015, even though she was coming back from an injury, she helped the US Women's national team win the World Cup. As Abby Wambach steps away from the US national team, Alex will become one of the team's leaders. Alex has great speed and athleticism, most likely from her days as a multi-sport athlete. Her opponents probably wish she had picked another sport to play, but she certainly made the best choice for all soccer fans.

17

Understand the Back Line

» *Defending*

It's good to have a general idea about what happens with the back line of your team during a game. This information will help you become a better player because you can fill in for players if they are out of position or help your teammates get to the right spot. Playing in the back line can be physically and mentally challenging because you have to concentrate on protecting your goalkeeper, throughout the entire game. In this book, we will talk about the defensive line as a back four that is made up of the following players: two center backs, one on the left and one on the right; a left back who plays in the wide defensive position on the left of the defense; and the right

The Back Line

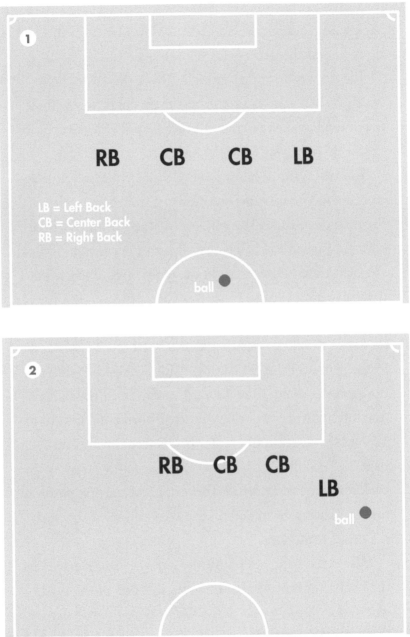

LB = Left Back
CB = Center Back
RB = Right Back

In #1 the ball is in the center of the field.
In #2 the ball is in the left defensive position.

back who plays in the wide defensive position on the right side of the defense (also known as "full backs").

The back four can never really cover the entire field width. When you watch the best teams play, you will see the defenders move together as a group and leave areas of the field open away from the ball.

You will want to know how to move your back line as a group, so you can cover as much of the entire width of the field as possible. We will look at the positions of the back four when the ball is played into the central midfield area, left defensive area, right defensive area, and central defensive area.

When the other team has the ball *in midfield*, your center backs should be positioned about 10 to 12 yards apart in the center of the field, just outside where the posts are positioned (about 10 to 15 yards away from the ball). The full backs should be on the same horizontal line 10 to 12 yards away from the center backs (see illustration 1, page 119). Skill 13 (page 103) discusses how far away the back four are from the ball. This is a good starting position for your back four to defend the goal and react to what the other team does.

When the ball goes out to the *left defensive position*, the back four move across to cover the side of the field where the danger is. The left back goes to the ball carrier to pressure the ball. The left center back covers at an angle

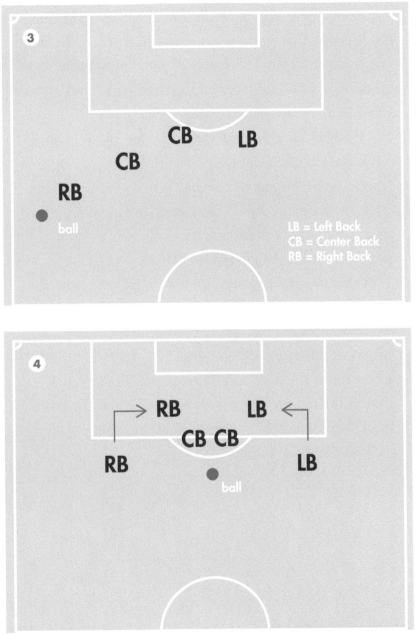

In #3 the ball is in the right defensive position.
In #4 the ball is in the central area of the goal.

of about 45 degrees about 10 yards away. The right center back gets in line with the left center back. Then, the right back gets in line and is around 10 yards away in the area between the penalty spot and the far post to "anchor" the back line (see illustration 2, page 119).

This leaves a big area of the field open, but if the ball is on your left side, there is no real threat on your right at this point in the game. If the ball goes out to your right side, the positions should be reversed, with the right back going out to the ball and the left back becoming the anchor (see illustration 3, page 121).

When the ball goes into the *central* area in front of your penalty box and your two central defenders have to go to pressure the ball and opponents in that tight space, your two full backs will drop back about 3 to 5 yards and come inside the field about 3 yards (see illustration 4, page 121). so they can cover the space behind the center backs and intercept any through-balls that get played behind the center backs.

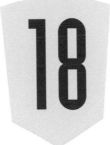
Cross the Ball

» *Passing*

One of the most exciting parts of the game for players, coaches, and fans is a cross into the area that creates a goal-scoring opportunity. Crossing the ball is not just about kicking it into the box and hoping the striker will put it in the goal. It's a complex skill that is easily learned and will help you become a better player.

When you are in position to cross the ball, you have one job, which is to put the ball into a space that helps your team score a goal. The best place to put the ball is in the space between the six-yard box and the penalty spot, called the "second six." If you cross the ball into the six-yard box, you increase the chances of the keeper catching

Crossing the Ball

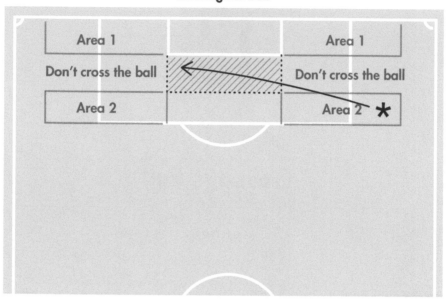

The shaded area is the second six—the target area for the ball.

In Area 1, cross the ball back away from the goal.
In Area 2, cross the ball into the second six, but keep the ball out of the six-yard box.

See ✱ for example.

the ball. If you cross the ball behind the second six, it becomes harder for your team to get a shot on the goal.

The technical focus for crossing should be on three things: (1) making good contact with the ball so it goes where you want it to go, (2) the angle of the cross as it passes through the second six, and (3) the height of the cross.

You won't want to cross the ball into the second six from the area at the side of the second six. Go past that space toward the goal line or put the cross in before you reach the second six. If your cross goes into the second six in a straight line, it's easier for the keeper to come and collect it or a defender to clear the ball.

The following are tips to help you decide which type of cross to make:

- If you go to the touchline and want to play the ball across the ground, use a *short-range pass* (page 26).

- If you get to the touchline and want to play the ball in the air, you are *chipping the ball* (page 39).

- If you cross the ball before the second six and you want to keep it on the ground, you are *bending the ball with the outside of the foot* (page 58) so it bends across the space in front of the keeper.

- If you cross the ball before the second six and you want the ball in the air, you are *chipping the ball* into the space.

When you learn to cross the ball, work on a good touch to make space for the cross. Get your head up, choose the type of cross you'll make, and make good contact with the ball.

To practice, start with the ball at your feet 25 yards out from the goal and 5 yards in from the touchline. Take two or three touches toward the goal line, and work on passing the ball through the second six. If you have some cones, mark this space out so you can monitor your progress. Think of the cross as a pass from the wing. This will help you stay focused on crossing the ball. Your job is to put the ball into the space. It's the striker's job to get into that space and get to the ball before the defender. Hit 20 balls from the right of the field, and then hit 20 balls from the left side of the field so you develop the skill with both feet.

When you are comfortable with this exercise, work on speeding up your approach and limiting your touches before you cross the ball. Fewer touches mean you can move faster because you won't have to break stride to touch the ball.

19

Defend the Cross

» *Defending*

When you defend crossed balls into the area, the first thing to consider is the position of your body when the ball comes into the 18-yard box. The best position is facing away from your goal and facing toward the top of the 18-yard box. If you can get your feet and body turned away from your own goal, it will help you avoid deflecting the ball into your own goal, which is obviously something you don't want to do. The best way to get your body facing the right way is to anticipate the danger before anyone else. To do this, you have to take up a position that allows you to see the following three things: (1) the player crossing the ball, (2) the player you are marking, and (3) the space where the ball will be going.

The best way to take up this spot is to turn your body so your shoulder is pointing toward the corner flag. Remember, keep your feet moving and keep looking over your shoulder. This allows you to see players who are in a wide position, the area behind or across the front of you that the attacking player is trying to get into, and your opponent. Watch the player crossing the ball. When this player's head goes down, this is the cue for you to get set to clear the ball. If you are facing away from the ball, you won't be in danger of deflecting the ball into your own goal or giving away a corner.

If you can't get your body facing the right way and you are facing your own goal, there are a few tips that can help, depending on what part of the penalty area you are in.

- **Outside of the near post (the area closer to the ball than the near post):** If you find yourself outside of the near post, try to clear the ball back and away over the area where the ball was crossed. If you can't get the ball away down the field, try to put it out for a throw, which allows your teammates to reorganize the defense and mark their opponents. If this isn't possible, get the ball out for a corner. Defending a corner still gives your team a chance to reorganize. Even though it's not a great spot to be in, it's better than not getting to the ball.

- **Outside of the far post (the area farther away from the ball than the far post):** If you are outside of the far post, don't clear the ball back across the goal. Try to help the ball on its way across the goal and away from danger. If you can't do this, get the ball out of play for a throw-in. If you can't get the ball out of play, put it out for a corner so your opponent's player at the far post doesn't get a chance on the ball. If they don't have a player back there, you can either let it go out of play or control it, turn away from your goal, and start your team's next attack.

- **In between the goal posts:** If you find yourself in front of your own goal and facing the net as the ball comes across, try to get to the ball first. Put the ball up in the air as high as you can. There's a good chance it will go out for a corner. You are in a tough spot, and getting the ball high up in the air is really the only option.

20

Create Space

» Passing » Running » Dribbling

There is a lot of space on the field, but the higher up the field you go (closer to the opponent's goal), the harder it is to find space because the other team will drop back and defend their goal. When you can't find space, you have to create space. The best soccer players create space for themselves and other players on their team using their movements and, sometimes, by not even moving at all.

There are a number of things you can do to create space. In all of these actions, the focus is on moving the other team's defenders and trying to get them to come out of their positions so they leave open space you can move into. You can do this in the following ways:

- Use quick, accurate passes to try to throw the defending team off-balance and confuse them, so you can open-up spaces on the field.

- Move away from the ball to open-up space.

- Dribble with the ball to bring defenders closer to the ball.

- Run with the ball at the defenders so they have to react to your movement.

Your coach will work with your team on these techniques, but here are some pointers so that you are ahead of the rest of the team.

You can use interpassing, which is a series of passes over different distances to move the other team around. A couple of short, accurate passes will bring them closer to the ball, and a longer pass gives you a chance to go into the spaces left by the players moving toward the ball. Some of these touches might be "one-touch" passes, so make sure you prepare your feet to do a one-touch pass and think about your pass to your teammate. If the pass is not to your teammate's feet, he or she probably can't make a one-touch pass. If the pass is too fast, an extra touch may be needed to control it and that will help the defenders.

Sometimes a simple movement across the face of a defender can create space. If the defender follows you, a gap opens up. If the defender doesn't, you might be in an open space. Stay on your toes and keep moving to help create space on the field.

There are times when you can create space for yourself and others just by holding the ball at your feet. If you can hold the ball for a few seconds, defenders will come toward you. Make sure you are sneaking a peek so you don't get caught with the ball. When players move toward you, you can either go into the space they just left or play a pass into that space to a supporting player. Have the confidence to try something different. Creativity is a great skill to have!

Dribbling at a single defender or running with the ball in open space will create space in other areas of the field. If no one comes to tackle you, keep going. If a player comes toward you, keep your head up and look for opportunities to pass the ball to an open player or beat that defender in a 1-vs.-1 situation.

As you can see, there are lots of ways you can create space for yourself and your teammates. The key to creating space lies in how you move when you have the ball and when you do not.

21

Break Their Lines

» *Passing* » *Running*

When you learn to break the line of your opponent, it will help you become a better soccer player. In every game, each team starts with a playing formation. There are many different formations, and you are probably familiar with many of them. Numbers are used to describe these formations. For example, 4-3-3 is four defenders, three midfielders, and three strikers; 4-4-2 is four defenders, four midfielders, and two strikers; 3-5-2 is three defenders, five midfielders, and two strikers; and 3-4-3 is three defenders, four midfielders, and three strikers.

Soccer players arrange themselves in lines that are similar to the numbers just mentioned: so, a back line of three

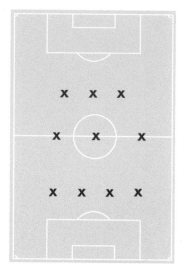

4-3-3

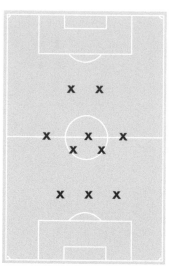

3-5-2

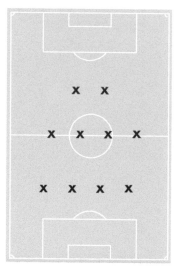

4-4-2

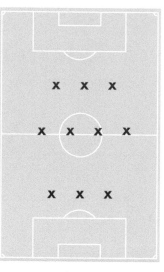

3-4-3

or four, a forward line of two or three, and midfield lines made up of two, three, four, or sometimes five players. The lines that the other team makes are the lines that you want to break.

Pretend these lines of players are connected by an invisible line (see illustrations). Your job is to get through these lines, and you can do this in the following three ways:

1. **Break their lines with a pass.** If you can break their forward line with a pass, you have the ball under control in midfield. This is a good position to be in because you can then start to break their lines in the midfield area and move the ball down the field. As you move down the field, your goal is to try to break their back line with a pass and get your players in behind their back four so you can create a chance to score a goal.

2. **Break their lines by running through with the ball.** This is an important skill for defenders to learn. When you break their striker's line by running with the ball, you become an extra midfielder. The key to playing successful soccer is getting more players around the ball than your opponent. Breaking the line with the ball will bring other defenders closer to you and open up spaces for your teammates to move into. This will be very frustrating to your opponents!

Breaking Lines

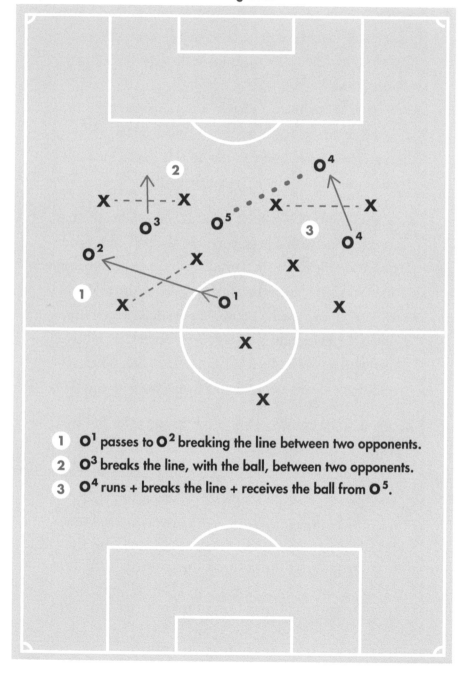

1. O^1 passes to O^2 breaking the line between two opponents.
2. O^3 breaks the line, with the ball, between two opponents.
3. O^4 runs + breaks the line + receives the ball from O^5.

3. **Break their lines with a supporting run.** This is simply making a run between two players from the other team in order to get into open space to receive a pass. When you make a run to break their back line, make sure you don't go offside, because then you can't get the ball.

There are more lines to break in midfield, so you can break lines going across the field to switch the play or just to keep possession. When you make runs to break lines, keep in mind where you are going and why. Simply running around the field won't help your team. Plan your runs so you support the player with the ball. You will become a better soccer player if you can master the skill of breaking lines with a pass, run, or the ball at your feet.

22

Live in the Triangle

» Passing

Another skill that follows from breaking lines is called "living in the triangle." When you are playing in a game your job is to get in between the defending, midfield, and attacking lines of the other team and take a supporting position to receive a pass from your teammate.

If you get too close to a defender or midfielder when you receive the ball, it is easy for the other team to figure out who is supposed to be marking you because the player nearest you will put you under pressure. Look for spaces between the other team's lines, which will create problems for your opponents. For example, if you can find a space between the central defender and the central midfielder

Live in the Triangle

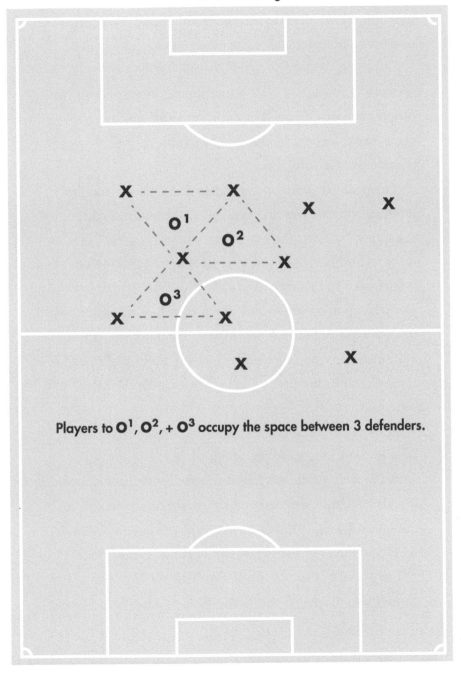

Players to O^1, O^2, + O^3 occupy the space between 3 defenders.

who may be 15 yards apart, the midfielder has to drop down to mark you, which opens up a space in midfield. Even better, the central defender may have to come forward to mark you, which then opens up a space in the other team's back line. If you can open up space in the other team's defensive line, and you help your team create possible scoring chances.

Teams don't move up and down the field in straight lines, so you can also find spaces in between the midfielders and in between the defenders. These are great positions to find because these players may not be sure who is supposed to be marking you. If they both come toward you when you get the ball, a quick pass to a teammate will open up spaces because two players are marking you. If neither player comes to mark you, you are in possession of the ball and unmarked, which is also a great position for your team.

How do you find these spaces in between their lines? Live in the triangle. When you look at the opposing team's players' positions, look for a group of three opposing players and imagine straight lines that connect them to make a triangle. When you see the triangle, fill that space and "live" in that space. By occupying that space, you will attract the attention of at least two of their players and maybe all three. This will be a big help to your team, and it also helps the player with the ball because it gives him or her a passing option.

When you have found the triangle and filled the space, look for spaces where you can play passes if you receive the ball and get your feet ready to receive the pass. Try not to stay in the space too long. The longer you stay in the space, the smaller it becomes, and the other team will react to your position. If you don't get the ball after a couple of seconds or the triangle starts to shrink, look for another triangle and move to that space. Keep moving and looking for triangles above the ball, and also below the ball because there are times when the ball can't go forward and the player in possession needs help.

SECRET

13

HYDRATE BEFORE THE GAME

To be ready to play, start drinking four hours before the game. Water is fine, but sports drinks with carbohydrates in them are better.

Cristiano Ronaldo

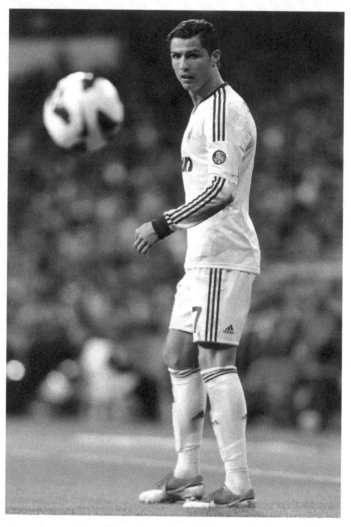

BORN: February 5, 1985 **POSITION:** Forward
TEAM: Real Madrid, Spain; Portugal national team

CRISTIANO RONALDO WASN'T THE FIRST "Ronaldo" in the sport of soccer. The first Ronaldo played for Brazil and won two World Cup titles. However, today, when we hear the name Ronaldo, we only think of the brilliant Portuguese attacker.

Ronaldo started his career in Portugal with his local club Nacional, but his potential was spotted very quickly by the great Portuguese club, Sporting. After 25 games, he was transferred to Manchester United where he became a soccer superstar, winning many honors including the Champions League in 2008. With the world at his feet, he left Manchester in 2009 and joined Real Madrid, where he became the highest paid player in history at that time. With Real Madrid, he continued to improve and helped the team win the Spanish title and the Champions League.

Ronaldo has played more than 100 times for his country. He is their all-time best goal scorer and has played in three World Cups and three European Championships for Portugal.

Ronaldo has great speed and power. He has worked very hard to develop his muscle strength, which helps him with the many 1-vs.-1 encounters he has in a game. Very often, he is too fast and too strong for his opponents, and he will just glide past them. If his opponents manage to slow him down, he uses his great skills and fast feet to get past them in tight spaces. In many games, he is almost impossible to stop. There is always more than one player trying to stop Ronaldo.

As with all great players, Ronaldo spends countless hours practicing his skills. He is known for taking amazing free kicks that bend and dip in the air. Practice makes perfect!

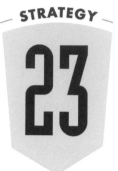

STRATEGY

23

What to Do 1 vs. 1

» *Running*

One of the most valuable skills you can learn and develop is beating a player in a 1-vs.-1 situation. The world's greatest players, such as Lionel Messi, Cristiano Ronaldo, and Alex Morgan, can beat players in 1-vs.-1 situations when it matters most.

The most important skill in this situation is confidence. The worst thing that can happen if you don't beat the player is that your team loses the ball. The other team will give it back to your team soon, so don't worry about losing the ball. Think about beating that player and creating a chance for your team. If you don't take the player on, you will never beat him or her. No one wins every 1 vs. 1, so just go for it!

There are two ways to beat a player in a 1-vs.-1 situation: with speed, if you have space, and with skill if you don't have the space.

When we talk about speed, we think of pure athletic speed or speed of thought, which is thinking about what you are going to do more quickly than your opponent can react. To use speed to beat a player, you need to first find or create space in order to get into a position to receive the ball. Your movement away from the ball will help you create space, and as the opposition reacts, you will attract a defender who is then isolated from his or her teammates.

Once you have space and the defender is isolated, you should start to look at the space you are going to get to, which will be the space behind the defender. As you receive the ball, have a touch to get the ball out of your feet, push the ball past the defender, and go into the space. Keep your body between the ball and the defender and use your body as a shield to stop the defender from getting the ball. Once you have pushed the ball into the open space past the defender, make sure you get the next touch on the ball, and you will have won that battle.

When you don't have a lot of space to work in, use your footwork to get yourself past the defender and try to throw the defender off-balance. Practice your favorite move as often as you can, and work on a backup trick in case the defender figures out what you are doing. Remember, confidence is the key to success and the more you try to take on the defender, the more you will beat him or her.

Keep your head up and make sure you can see the ball and the defender you are playing against. Also make sure your body is opened up so you can receive the ball in a good position. Get your first touch on the ball and out of your feet so you have room to move and beat the player with your trick. Keep your body low and your knees bent so you can move easily from side to side, and use your body as a shield, positioning yourself between the ball and the player.

SECRET 14

HYDRATE DURING THE GAME

Make sure you bring fluids to drink during the game. Drink 6 to 12 ounces every 15 minutes to stay hydrated. Write your name on your bottle.

24

Get the Ball Back

» Defending

When your team loses possession of the ball, the focus should change to winning the ball back as quickly as possible. Often, players who are not positioned as a defender or defensive midfielder don't realize the needed change in focus, and, very quickly, the team is under pressure and defending its goal. In soccer games today, players need to think about not only their position on the team but also about their roles on the team when in and out of possession of the ball. When your team doesn't have the ball, your coach will want you to do everything possible to win the ball back!

There are many skills you will learn as a defender, and here are a few examples.

- **Defending a player with the ball who has his or her back to you.** The first thing to do is get into position behind the attacker in a space where you can see the ball. If you can't see the ball, you are guessing, and you could guess wrong. Defenders can't guess. They have to know where the ball is. Get nice and low so you can react to the ball carrier's movement, but don't put too much weight on one foot because you will become off-balanced. For example, this makes it difficult to push off to the right if all your weight is on your right foot. Also avoid making contact with the ball carrier. If you do, he or she knows where you are and can make a better decision. Make him or her guess where you are or, better still, make him or her look for you and take his or her eye off the ball. Stay in this position and delay the player. Don't let the player turn by matching his or her movement, and if the player has to hold the ball for longer than three or four seconds, there is a good chance you can get help from a teammate.

- **Open play in midfield.** Your focus is to decide if you can win the ball in a tackle. If you are late in the tackle, it will be a foul, and you may receive a yellow or red card, which certainly won't help your team. If you can't make a tackle, stay on your feet and get in a defensive position with your shoulder facing the ball carrier and your knees bent so you are balanced. In open play in the midfield area, there is always help close by, so do not jump in at the ball and miss. Your coach may call this "diving in." Be patient. Keep your eye on the ball and stop the ball carrier from going forward, if possible. If the ball carrier pushes the ball out in front, this is your chance to step into the space between the carrier and the ball and win it!

- **A 1-vs.-1 situation out on the wings.** Your main job is to delay the player with the ball and not get beat. Get your feet in the right place and point your shoulders at the ball carrier. Take control of the situation and force the player where you want to go. Stay on your feet, focus on the ball, and when the player tries a trick, *react to the ball instead of the player's body movement*. Good defenders are patient, focused, and a huge asset to any team.

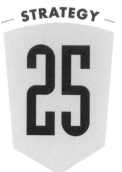

STRATEGY

25

Work Together on the Back Line

» *Defending*

As you learned earlier, the back four work together to cover the field from side to side. It's also good to know what everyone's job is on the field so you can help out when needed. The more versatile you are as a player, the more important you become to your coach and team. Of course, you will make mistakes, so remember that you are still learning the game, and you can learn from your mistakes.

Let's now look at how the back four move together as a group up and down the field. As a rule, the back four work together between your own penalty area and the halfway line. They don't want to drop back into the penalty area if they don't have to, because that makes it harder for the keeper to see the ball. If possible, they want to hold their line at the edge of the penalty area. As the team moves forward, the back four should stay together on a horizontal line up to the halfway line. The full backs, or even one of the center backs, may venture forward to help in attack, but the halfway line is your "base camp" when your team is attacking.

If you are playing in the back line, you should always look for cues to tell you how to move up, how to drop back, and to where. For example, if the midfielders or strikers are able to put pressure on the player with the ball, the back four can be about 10 yards behind the midfielders so you can squeeze the other team back and take away their space. As you continue to squeeze your opponent back, your back four can move as far forward as the halfway line as long as pressure is kept on the ball carrier.

When the other team gets free and the player on the ball has time to look forward and pass, the back four should be ready to retreat as a group. Look at the player on the ball and look for the cues. If the player opens his or her hips up and tries to hit a long ball into the space behind the back four, move back toward your goal right away so you take the space away. It's important that the back four move together so they can defend as a group.

Don't worry about the player in front of you. If you see the cue for the long ball, go back, and then you can reset and get ready to defend. This tactic is much easier than chasing the player after the ball has gone over your head.

If the player on the ball breaks free and starts running with the ball, the back four should start to retreat and take away the space behind them. In this case, if the ball carrier isn't challenged, the back four can retreat only so far. As a rule, they would hold on the edge of the penalty area and not drop back any farther. If the ball carrier stops going forward and turns back, the back four should start to move forward so the process of winning the ball is started.

SECRET

15

BE PATIENT

Remember, you are learning the game and it takes time for any back four to become solid and strong. Be patient, learn from the mistakes you make, and listen to your coach's instructions.

26

Get to the Arriving Triangle

» Running » Shooting

To "finish a cross," the three main things to focus on are the following: arriving in a position to score, getting to the ball first, and hitting the target.

There are three areas coaches want you to get into, and some coaches call this "the arriving triangle" (see the illustration on page 154). These areas are the near post, far post, and central area of the goal. Whichever space you decide to fill, it's important that your run into that space isn't in a straight line or at the same pace, as these tactics will make it easier for the defenders to mark you. Accelerate into the space later in the run so you can separate

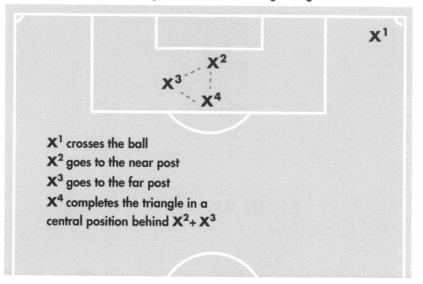

X^1 crosses the ball
X^2 goes to the near post
X^3 goes to the far post
X^4 completes the triangle in a
central position behind $X^2 + X^3$

yourself from the defender who is marking you. If you sprint too soon, you risk getting into the space too early or allowing the defender to catch you as you slow down. Try to make your run in a diagonal line so you can see the player crossing the ball. This means that you read the cues he or she is sending you and have a good idea of when the ball is going to be crossed. You can also change the angle and direction of your run. If you can do this, it may unbalance or confuse the defender and give you a chance to get the separation you need. Be creative!

If you make a run to the near post, try to get to the outside of the defender. This means you are closer to the ball than the defender, and this will help you get to the ball first. It's also important to try to stay inside the goal post with your run. This will also help you hit the target. If you pass the post toward the edge of the six-yard box, it becomes harder to hit the target because you have to turn your body as you connect with the ball. Keep things simple and give yourself the best chance to succeed.

If you make a run to the far post, try again to get the inside line of the defender and look for a position either in-line with the far post or just outside of it. Try to stay in the space between the edge of the six-yard box and the goal post. As you get into position, make sure that you are not in a horizontal line with the player in the near-post area so you increase your chances of getting to the ball. If you are on the same line and if the ball misses the opposing player, it will most likely miss you too!

With both the near-post and far-post runs, try to stay in the "second six" because the keeper will most likely be in the six-yard box and any contact with the keeper could be a foul.

If you go into the center of the goal, try to find a space just behind the penalty spot and behind the players in the near- and far-post areas so you provide another option for the player crossing the ball. This also covers the area, in case the defending team gets a touch on the ball first. If you are in this spot, you can pick the ball up and shoot.

27

Get Ready to Score

» *Passing* » *Shooting*

After you get into the "arriving triangle," you'll need to know what to do next. It is very important to get the first touch on the ball as the cross comes into the goal area. In the near-post area, if the ball comes from the right, use your right foot to connect with the ball. If you let it come across your body, you give the defender more time to intercept or block the ball. If the ball comes from the left, use your left foot to connect, so you have a better chance of first contact.

In the far-post area, get your body set, be on your toes, and be ready for the ball. You will have a little more time than the player at the near post, so make good use of that time. Breathe and relax, so if the ball does come to you, you are ready for action. If you are stiff and tense, you won't make the best contact with the ball.

In the central area, get set and face the goal. In this space, you may have to deal with the ball being deflected by another player or you may intercept a clearance by the defenders. Here, you need to be on your toes and ready to react to any situation.

The last piece of the puzzle is hitting the target and making the keeper save the ball. In the near-post area, you are trying to deflect the ball toward the goal, rather than smash it through the goal. You want to use the pace of the cross and change the direction of the ball toward the goal. Sometimes just getting your toe to the ball will do the job, but the best surface to use is the inside of your foot. Concentrate on trying to keep the ball low so it's hard for the keeper to make a save and follow the ball after you hit it, in case there is a rebound. If the ball goes past you, get ready for another chance because the ball is still in a "dangerous" area of the field.

At the back post, you will want to pass the ball into the goal using the side of your foot so you have a better chance of an accurate strike. Always try to place the ball into the far corner of the goal because the keeper will have to change direction to make a save, making the goal harder to stop. In this position, try to make a good contact, first-time shot if possible, but if you think you have time, settle the ball and pass it into the goal.

In the central area, your focus is on getting prepared to hit the target if the ball comes to you directly, as well as intercepting attempted clearances and then hitting the target. As with the player at the far post, get to your spot, face the goal, and relax so you are ready to act. If you can shoot side-footed the first time, that is the best option. If not, settle the ball, focus on making good contact with the ball, and be ready in case it comes back out again.

The ball won't always come your way, but keep making the runs to fill the spaces so you are in position to score when it does come into your space.

FOR
PARENTS

FOR PARENTS

Thank you for choosing this book. As parents, you want to help your kids improve their soccer game, excel in the sport, and enjoy playing. Parents have a very important role in their children's success: to always be a positive soccer parent.

What Is Success?

In a professional soccer game, it's easy to define success: Who won? We don't even care why or how they won. The team may have won the ugliest game you have ever seen. They could have had shots that hit the post and crossbar and three goals called back, but all that really matters is the final score. In youth soccer, defining success is much harder.

If the score of the game was the defining factor in success in youth soccer, 50 percent of players and coaches would fail. If results are used to determine success, only one team from each division each year would "succeed," and the rest of the teams would fail. Clearly, it is not a good idea to use scores or results to determine success in youth soccer.

Here are some questions to consider:

- Is your child having fun? Do you see smiles and hear laughter?

- Does your child respect the rules of the game and understand that winning and losing are part of the game?

- Is your child staying fit and healthy and getting exercise from the sport?

- Is your child making new friendships and growing his or her social network from playing soccer?

- Is your child learning new skills?

- Does your child plan to play next season?

If the answer to these questions is "yes," your child is successful in soccer!

Encourage Practice

Author Malcolm Gladwell, in his book *Outliers: The Story of Success*, stated that 10,000 hours is the magic number of practice hours to reach an expert level of performance. This concept, known as the 10,000-hour rule, has become controversial, particularly in the world of sports. It's now recognized that the quality of practice is most important.

If you want to help your child reach his or her maximum potential as a soccer player, encourage practice whenever there is free time. Children can practice independently many of the skills and strategies featured in this book. This gives them ownership of their development and lets them accelerate at their own pace.

As little as 20 minutes of practice three times a week will make a big difference in children's soccer skills and help them become better players. Hard work is the key to success, and talent is heavily linked with hard work and dedication. Talented expert performers, whether in the world of sports or entertainment, have a great work ethic and do practice harder and longer than their less-talented counterparts.

You will be pleased to learn that work ethics can be transferred to school-work as well!

The Role You Play

If you have watched your child play in soccer games, you have probably seen the "crazy soccer parent" running up and down the line, screaming out advice, berating the officials, second-guessing the coaches, criticizing the players, and embarrassing their child. I have seen many of these parents, and I believe these parents do think they are helping the team and their child.

Shouting instructions onto the field is like having a parent at the back of a ninth-grade math class shouting out, "Divide it first! Now subtract it! Don't add it!" A soccer game is an extension of practice sessions, and the players will only learn if they are given the opportunity to fail and then learn from their mistakes.

Your job is to support your child's development in soccer and not push to accelerate it. All children develop at different paces, and they will all excel in due time. You get to see them through the journey. One of the best things about team sports is the friendships made along the way. The "crazy soccer parent" invariably spoils this for the child. It's not uncommon for players to be cut from youth teams because the baggage the parents bring along is too disruptive and detrimental.

Remember, it's their team and their experience. Behave like a guest, support your child, and enjoy watching them play.

At the Game

For a soccer player, there is nothing better than hearing people cheer for you or your team. When you watch your child play, cheer! Offer encouragement rather than advice. Soccer games do not have time-outs, so there is very little a coach can do to change what happens in a game when the whistle blows. Coaches want their players to make their own decisions based on what they see and their knowledge of the game. The younger the players are, the harder it is for them to make decisions. At times, they may appear confused. Many parents, and some coaches, see this as an opportunity to "help" the players and shout out instructions.

However, by the time a parent has shouted an instruction, the picture will have changed on the field. There are lots of moving parts in the game of soccer, and the picture changes quickly. If children try to follow their parents' instructions, it will most likely result in them losing the ball through no fault of their own. Also, this type of support won't help young soccer players in the long term, because they will wait for the instructions and not learn to make their own decisions. Instead, celebrate the good plays and your child's hard work and contributions to the team.

Showing Support

The game is over. You are on the way home, and you want to talk about the game. What should you say and how do you start the conversation?

As a parent, the five golden words you should begin with are, "I love watching you play!" It doesn't matter what the score was or how the team played. What matters is that you got to spend time with your child. Here are some examples of questions to get the conversation started:

- What did you think of the game?

- What were you thinking about at half-time? What were you thinking about in the last few minutes of the game (if it was a tense and exciting game)?

- Who do you think played well on your team?

- What do you think was your best part of the game?

- What did your coach say after the game?

- How is your team preparing for the next game? What can your team do better next time?

This is a better way to talk about the game than a post-game critique of the team, officials, and any poor decisions you feel the coaches made. Remember to compliment the other team so your child learns it's important to respect the opponent.

A vital skill for soccer players is the ability to self-reflect. By engaging children in these types of discussions, you are helping them build critical-thinking skills that will also serve them well in other areas of their lives.

ACKNOWLEDGMENTS

To the best team, the home team, my family: Joanne, Hope, Ollie, Jake, and Lawrence. Family isn't everything—it's the only thing.

This book is dedicated to every player and coach I have had the opportunity to work with. You made me a better coach and I am grateful for that. There isn't enough space to name you all but you know who you are!

Many years ago a great coach, Roy Rees, turned on a light in my brain and it continues to burn bright. Thanks, Roy!

INDEX

A

Above the ball, 15
Arriving triangle, 156
  getting to, 153–155
Attack, 15

B

Back four, 15, 150
Back line, 133, 135
  understanding the,
    118–122
  working together
    on the, 150–152
Ball
  above the, 15
  avoiding running
    of, 92
  beating player
    without
    touching,
    103–104
  below the, 15
  bending of
    inside, 36–38
    outside, 58–60
  breaking lines by
    running through
    with the, 135
  chipping the,
    39–41, 125
  crossing the,
    123–126
  finding space
    behind the, 71

getting back,
  147–149
getting behind the,
  81–83
helping player on
  the, 109–112
juggling the, 48–49
keeping or passing,
  93–95
making throw-in
  with, 86–87
manipulation of, 50
possession of the,
  105
receiving the,
  20–21
receiving
  thrown-in, 88–89
shielding the,
  46–47
spinning the, 58–60
striking on a volley,
  42–43
using thighs
  and chest in
  controlling,
  24–25
Beckham, David,
  32–33
Below the ball, 15
Bending the ball
  inside, 58–60
  with inside of the
    foot, 125

outside, 36–38
Box, shooting from
  the inside of,
  52–53
Breakaway, 15
Breaking lines,
  133–137
Break the line, 15

C

Carbohydrates, 108
  replacing, 104
Center backs, 14
Chest, using your,
  24–25
Chipping the ball,
  39–41, 125
  rear view of, 41
  side view of, 40
Closed space, 16
Clothing, wearing
  proper, 89
Coaches, 8, 10, 164
  helping, 158
Confidence, 52,
  144–145
Control, 15
Cool down, 28
Corners, 17, 36
Creating space,
  130–132
Cross
  defending the,
    127–129

finishing a, 153
Crossbar challenge, 41
Crossing the ball, 123–126
Cues, 15

D
Defender, 12, 13, 14
  shielding the ball and, 46–47

Defending, 18
  back line in, 118–122
  cross, 127–129
  getting ball back in, 147–149
  getting behind the ball in, 81–83
  helping team in, 113–115
  learning by watching in, 64–66
  pattern recognition in, 90–92
  receiving throw-in in, 88–89
  wide positions in, 78–80
  working together on the back line in, 150–152
Directional pass, 105–106
Down low, 16
Down the field, 15
Dribbling, 18
  beating player without touching ball in, 103–104

keeping or passing ball in, 93–95
playing with both feet, 50–51
spatial awareness in, 130–132
Drills, 25, 41, 69, 74, 126
Drop down, 15

E
Elecrolytes, replacing, 104

F
Far post, 16, 156–157
Feet, playing with both, 50–51
Field, 16–17
First attacker, 109
First defender, 113, 114–115
Forward (attacker), 12, 13
  Hamm, Mia, as, 84–85
  Messi, Lionel, as, 96–97
  Morgan, Alex, as, 116–117
  Ronaldo, Cristiano, as, 142–143
  Sinclair, Christine, as, 56–57
Forward line, 135
Foul, 17
Free kicks, 17, 36, 39, 92
Front foot, 16
  receiving the ball on the, 23
Full backs, 14, 120, 151

G
Game
  parents at the, 164–165
  rehydrating after, 104
  showing respect for, 23
Gladwell, Malcolm, 162
Goalkeeper (keeper/goalie), 13, 14
  shooting against the, 54–55
  working with, 12, 14
Goal kick, 18
Goal line, 51
Goals, 17
  setting your, 141

H
Half backs, 14
Half turned, 22
Half volley, striking the ball on the, 42, 43
Hamm, Mia, 84–85
Heading the ball, 61–62
Heavy pass, 16
Higher up the field, 16
Hydration, 104, 112, 141, 146

I
Instep pass, 30

J
Juggling the ball, 48–49

K

Keeping or passing
the ball, 93–95
Kicks
free, 17, 36, 39, 92
goal, 18
left-footed, 37
penalty, 18
right-footed, 37

L

Learning by watching,
64–66
Left-footed kicks, 37
Light pass, 16
Lines, breaking their,
133–137
Live games, watching,
60
Living in the triangle,
138–141
Long-distance passes,
34–35
Low down, 16

M

Marking, 16
Messi, Lionel, 96–97,
144
Midfielder, 13–14, 66
Beckham, David,
as, 32–33
Sinclair, Christine
as, 56–57
Midfield lines, 135
Midfield, open play
in, 148–149
Mid-range passes,
29–31, 35
Morgan, Alex,
116–117, 144

N

Notes, taking, 38, 65
Nutrition, 108

O

Offside, 18
Offside rule, 75
One-touch pass, 16
1-vs.-1 situations,
114, 144–145,
149
Opened up, 22
Open space, 17, 39
*Outliers: The Story of
Success*
(Gladwell), 162

P

Parents
defining of success
and, 160–162
encouraging
practice, 162
at the game,
164–165
role of, 163–164
showing support,
165–166
Pass
choosing right,
105–108
directional,
105–106
light, 16
possession, 106
receiving a, 22–23,
73–74
short-range, 125
side-foot, 29
taking risks with,
107–108
Passing, 18
beating player
without touching
ball in, 103–104
bending the ball in
inside, 58–60
outside, 36–38

breaking lines in,
133–137
chipping the ball
in, 39–41
choosing right pass
in, 105–106
crossing the ball in,
123–126
getting past the
other team in,
98–102
getting ready
to score in,
156–158
heading the ball in,
61–62
helping player
on the ball in,
109–112
keeping ball in,
93–95
long-distance,
34–35
making throw-in
in, 86–87
mid-range, 29–31
pattern recognition
in, 67–69, 90–92
receiving a pass in,
22–23
receiving the ball
in, 20–21
receiving throw-in
in, 88–89
shooting against
the keeper in,
54–55
short-range, 26–28
spatial awareness
in, 130–132
striking on a volley,
42–43
wide positions in,
78–80

Patience, 152
Pattern juggling, 48, 49
Pattern recognition, 67–69, 90–92
Penalty, taking a, 44–45
Penalty kick, 18
Physical ability, 9
Play, 17–18
Players
  beating, without touching ball, 103–104
  helping on the ball, 109–112
Playing formations, 133
Playing with both feet, 50–51
Positions, 12–14
Possession pass, 106
Practice
  encouraging, 162
  preparing for, 102, 115
Psychological skills, 9

R
Readiness to score, 156–158
Right-footed kicks, 37
Role model, picking a, 49
Ronaldo, Cristiano, 142–143, 144
Running, 18
  beating player without touching ball in, 103–104
  breaking lines in, 133–137

getting to arriving triangle in, 153–155
keeping or passing ball in, 93–95
spatial awareness in, 70–72, 130–132
staying outside in, 75–77
wide positions in, 78–80

S
Safe space, 17, 20
Score, getting ready to, 156–158
Second attacker, 109
Second defender, 113
Second six, 123, 124
Self-reflection, 166
Shielding the ball, 46–47
Shoes, wearing proper, 89
Shooting
  bending the ball inside in, 58–60
  outside in, 36–38
  chipping the ball in, 39–41
  getting ready to score in, 156–158
  getting to arriving triangle in, 153–155
  heading the ball in, 61–62
  from inside the box in, 52–53
  against the keeper in, 54–55
  taking a penalty in, 44–45

Short-range passes, 26–28, 115, 125
Side foot, in making short-range passes, 26–28
Side-foot pass, 29
Side on, 22
Side-to-side movements, 51
Sinclair, Christine, 56–57
Skills
  bending the ball inside, 58–60
  outside, 36–38
  chipping the ball, 39–41
  heading the ball, 61–62
  juggling the ball, 48–49
  long-distance passes, 34–35
  mid-range passes, 29–31
  playing with both feet, 50–51
  receiving the ball, 20–21
  receiving the pass, 22–23
  shielding the ball, 46–47
  shooting against the keeper, 54–55
  shooting from inside the box, 52–53
  short-range passes, 26–28
  striking on a volley, 42–43
  taking a penalty, 44–45

171

using thighs and chest, 24–25
Soccer terms, 15–18
Spatial awareness, 70–72, 130–132
Spinning, 36
  clockwise, 37, 58
  counter-clockwise, 37, 58
Staying onside, 75–77
Straight juggling, 48, 49
Strategies
  beating player without touching the ball, 103–104
  being aware of your space, 70–72
  breaking lines, 133–137
  choosing right pass, 105–108
  creating space, 130–132
  crossing the ball, 123–126
  defending the cross, 127–129
  getting ball back, 147–149
  getting behind the ball, 81–83
  getting past other team, 98–102
  getting ready to score, 156–158
  getting to arriving triangle, 153–155
  helping player on the ball, 109–112
  helping team defend, 113–115

keeping or passing the ball, 93–95
learning by watching, 64–66
living in the triangle, 138–141
making a throw-in, 86–87
1-vs.-1 situations, 144–145, 149
pattern recognition, 67–69, 90–92
receiving a pass, 73–74
receiving a throw-in, 88–89
staying onside, 75–77
understanding the back line, 118–122
wide positions in, 78–80
working together on back line, 150–152
Striking on a volley, 42–43
Success, defining, 160–162
Support, 16
  showing, 165–166
Supporting run, breaking their lines with a, 137
Sweepers, 14

T
Tactical understanding, 9
Team
  getting ball past other, 98–102

helping with defense, 113–115
Team player, being a, 112
Technical ability, 9
Thighs, using your, 24–25
Third attacker, 109
Throw-in, 18
  receiving, 88–89
  taking a, 86–87
Triangle
  arriving, 153–155, 156
  living in the, 138–141

U
Under pressure, 16
Understanding the back line, 118–122

V
Volley, striking on a, 42–43

W
Watching, learning by, 64–66
Wide positions, 65, 78–80
Wing backs, 14
Women's soccer, 85
Work ethics, 162
Working together on back line, 150–152
World Cup, 8, 10, 33, 117

SECRETS: DID YOU FIND THEM ALL?

1 Respect the Game 23

2 Cool Down 28

3 Take Notes 38

4 Pick a Role Model 49

5 Watch Live Games 60

6 Stay in Shape 83

7 Wear the Proper Shoes and Clothing 89

8 Prepare for Practice 102

9 Rehydrate after the Game 104

10 Eat to Succeed 108

11 Be a Team Player 112

12 Prepare for Practice 115

13 Hydrate before the Game 141

14 Hydrate during the Game 146

15 Be Patient 152

16 Help Your Coach 158

CPSIA information can be obtained
at www.ICGtesting.com
Printed in the USA
BVHW060950230919
559149BV00023B/1436/P